THE VEGAN COOKBOOK

50 DINNER RECIPES

VIRGINIA FARMVILLE

TABLE OF CONTENTS

SWEET CORN AND ZUCCHINIS RATATOUILLE

A delicious healthy vegetable packed ratatouille by Curtis Stone. Great as a side dish!

MAKES 8 SERVING/ TOTAL TIME 25 MINUTE

INGREDIENTS

3 tablespoons olive oil

2 small red onions, medium dice

4 garlic cloves, finely chopped

2 red capsicum, medium dice

2 green capsicum, medium dice

6 **zucchinis**, medium dice, green parts only

4 ears fresh yellow sweet corn, husk removed (about 3 cups of kernels)

1/2 cup fresh parsley, finely chopped

4 tablespoons fresh thyme, chopped

1/2 cup basil leaves, finely chopped

4 tablespoons fresh lemon juice

METHOD

STEP 1

Heat the oil in a large saucepot over medium-high heat.

STEP 2

Add the onions and saute for about 4 minutes or until slightly softened.

STEP 3

Add the garlic and saute for about 30 seconds or until fragrant.

STEP 4

Add the red and green capsicum and saute for about 4 minutes or until slightly softened.

STEP 5

Add the zucchinis and corn and saute for about 5 minutes or until they are crisp-tender.

STEP 6

Stir in the parsley, thyme, basil leaves and lemon juice.

STEP 7

Season to taste with salt and pepper and serve.

NUTRITION VALUE

615 KJ Energy, 6.3g fat, 1g saturated fat, 4.7g fiber, 4.7g protein, 22.4g carbs.

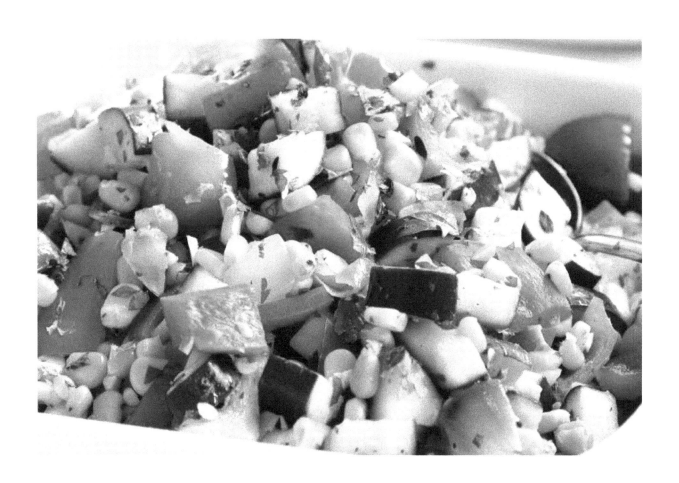

ZUCCHINIS 'NOODLE' SALAD WITH THAI CORIANDER PESTO

Strips of zucchinis make a great substitute for noodles in this **vegan-friendly** picnic idea by Dani Venn.

MAKES 5 **SERVING**/ **TOTAL** TIME 20 **MINUTE**

INGREDIENTS

4 medium-sized **zucchinis**, ends trimmed

2 cups coriander (stalks and leaves), washed, roughly chopped

1/2 cup raw macadamia nuts, plus a few for garnish

1 stalk fresh lemongrass, finely diced (about 1 tablespoon)

1/2 long red chili, seeded, chopped

1 fresh kaffir lime leaf, finely sliced (or bottled)

1/4 cup melted coconut oil

1 teaspoon chopped garlic

Juice of 1 lime

100g cherry tomatoes

METHOD

STEP 1

To make the zucchinis noodles use a mandolin with a julienne attachment and slice into 2cm thick noodles, alternatively, cut zucchinis into 2cm wide strips and julienne into thin strips. Set aside in mixing bowl.

STEP 2

To make coriander pesto place coriander, macadamia nuts, lemongrass, chili, kaffir lime leaf, coconut oil and garlic, into a small mixer or blender, and blend until a smooth consistency is achieved. Taste and season with a little sea salt and about a teaspoon of lime juice.

STEP 3

When ready to serve, add 4 tablespoons of pesto to the zucchinis and mix well. Add tomatoes and garnish with extra chopped macadamias. Serve as part of a shared picnic.

NUTRITION VALUE

1190 KJ Energy, 8.7g fat, 1.9g saturated fat, 13.6g fiber, 11.3g protein, 32.2g carbs.

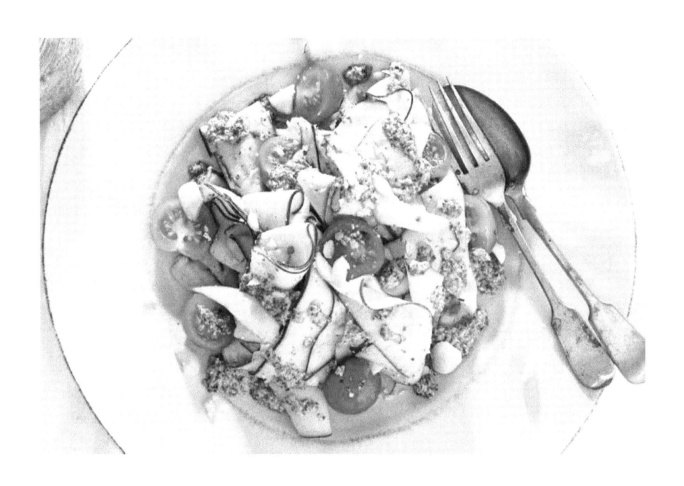

SUGAR SNAP PEA SALAD WITH SHAVED ONION, RADISH, BASIL, AND MINT

Follow directions for blanching snap peas, and you'll never serve a leathery or mushy green again.

MAKES 8 SERVING/ TOTAL TIME 25 MINUTE

INGREDIENTS

680g sugar snap peas, trimmed, strings removed

4 radishes, trimmed

1/3 cup extra-virgin olive oil

1/4 cup fresh lemon juice

Sea salt

2 cups (not packed) rocket

3/4 cup (about 1 small-medium) very thinly sliced white onion

1/2 cup (not packed) fresh small basil leaves

1/2 cup (not packed) fresh small mint leaves

METHOD

STEP 1

In a large saucepan of boiling salted water over high heat, cook the sugar snap peas for about 1 minute, or until crisp-tender. Drain. Rinse with cold water; drain well. Pat dry. Cut the pea pods in half lengthwise, leaving the peas attached on each side of the pods. Set the pea pods aside to drain.

STEP 2

cut the radishes into paper-thin slices. Cover with plastic wrap and refrigerate until cold. Drain the radishes well before tossing them in the salad.

STEP 3

Season the salad with salt and serve immediately.

NUTRITION VALUE	397 KJ Energy, 7g fat, 1.1g saturated fat, 2.4g fiber, 2.3g protein, 6.7g carbs.

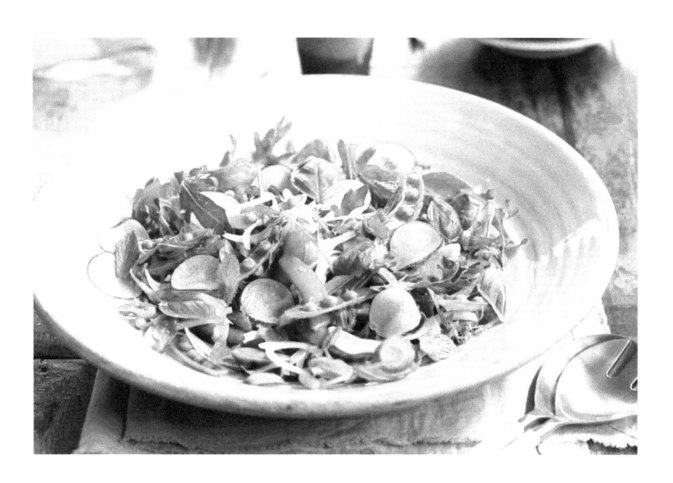

GREEN BEAN GRATIN WITH CHERRY TOMATO CONFIT AND MACADAMIA NUTS

A quick and delicious green bean gratin recipe with a zesty finish!

INGREDIENTS

30g of baguette, cut into 4 pieces

1/2 cup macadamia nuts

700g green beans, ends trimmed, cut diagonally in half crosswise

1 tablespoon olive oil

2 medium shallots, sliced about (3/4 cup)

2 tablespoons baby capers

1 1/2 teaspoons fine lemon zest

1/3 cup extra-virgin olive oil

2 tablespoons fresh lemon juice

2 punnets (500g) cherry tomatoes, halved

1 tablespoon finely chopped fresh flat-leaf parsley

METHOD

STEP 1

Preheat oven to 190◦C (170◦C fan). In a food processor, pulse the bread to fine crumbs. Reserve 1/2 cup of breadcrumbs on a large baking tray and discard any remaining crumbs. Pulse the nuts for 10 seconds, or to fine crumbs. Mix bread crumbs and nuts on baking tray then toast them in the oven, stirring occasionally, for about 8 minutes, or until golden. Set aside.

STEP 2

.Add the beans and cook for 4 minutes, or until bright green and just tender. Drain and place beans in large bowl of iced water to cool completely. Drain well, pat beans dry then place in a large bowl.

STEP 3

Add the capers and lemon zest and cook for 2 minutes, or until heated through and fragrant. Stir in the extra-virgin olive oil and lemon juice.

NUTRITION VALUE

870 KJ Energy, 16.9g fat, 2.5g saturated fat, 4.7g fiber, 3.6g protein, 14.5g carbs.

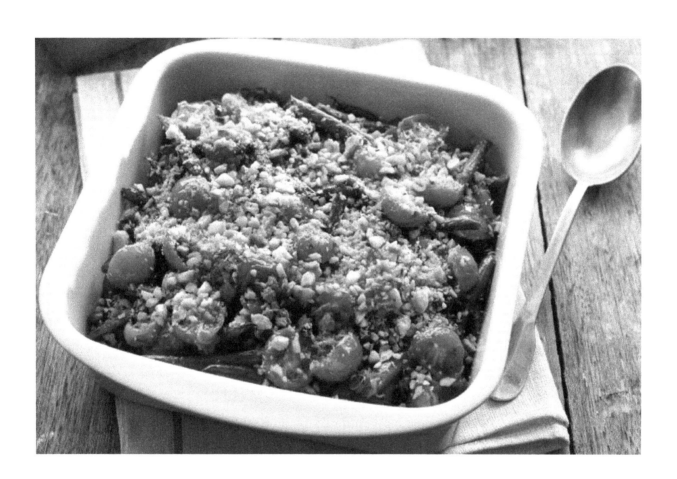

KALE, QUINOA AND ROASTED PUMPKIN PILAF

This hearty **vegan** pilaf combines sweet pumpkin, crunchy pepitas and healthy kale with spice-filled quinoa.

MAKES 4 SERVING/ TOTAL TIME 30 MINUTE

INGREDIENTS

800g **pumpkin**, peeled, seeded, cut into 1.5cm cubes

Spray olive oil

1 tablespoon olive oil

1 onion, finely chopped

2 garlic cloves, crushed

1 teaspoon finely grated ginger

1 teaspoon ground coriander

1/2 teaspoon ground turmeric

190g (1 cup) quinoa, rinsed, drained

100g Coles Chopped Kale

40g (1/4 cup) pepitas

Salt, to season

METHOD

STEP 1

Preheat oven to 200°C or 180°C fan forced. Line a large baking tray with baking paper. Place the pumpkin on prepared tray, spray with olive oil. Roast for 30 - 40 minutes or until golden and tender.

STEP 2

Meanwhile, heat the oil in a large saucepan over a medium heat. Cook onion, stirring occasionally for 5 minutes or until softened. Add the garlic, ginger, coriander and turmeric, cook stirring for 1 minute.

STEP 3

Add quinoa and 500ml (2 cups) water, bring to the boil. Reduce heat to low, cover and simmer for 12-15 minutes, or until water has evaporated and quinoa is al dente. Stir through kale until just wilted, then gently stir through the roasted pumpkin, pepitas and season with salt and freshly ground black pepper.

NUTRITION VALUE

1560 KJ Energy, 14g fat, 2.5g saturated fat, 8.5g fiber, 14g protein, 50g carbs.

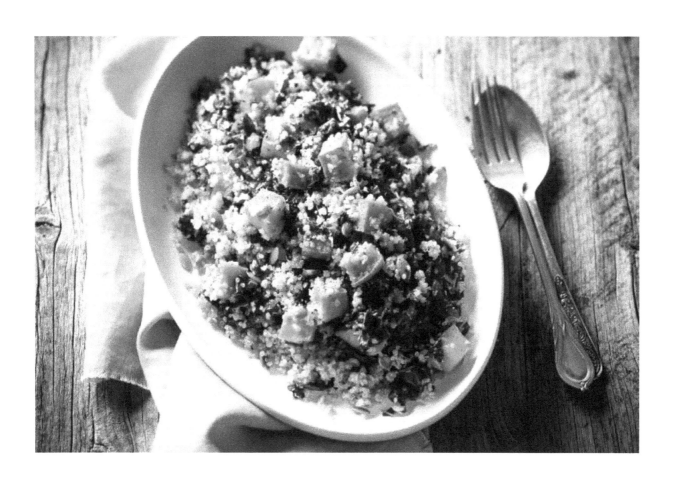

MARINATED ARTICHOKE AND CANNELLINI BEAN SALAD

This **vegan**-friendly salad combines the texture and flavors of artichoke and cannellini beans with the crunch of pine nuts.

MAKES 4 SERVING/ TOTAL TIME 4 MINUTE

INGREDIENTS

340g jar marinated artichoke hearts (see note)

400g can cannellini beans, drained, rinsed

2 tablespoons pine nuts, toasted

1 bunch rocket

2 tablespoons lemon juice

1/4 cup small fresh flat-leaf parsley leaves

METHOD

STEP 1

Drain artichokes, reserving 1 tablespoon of the marinade.

STEP 2

Heat a greased chargrill pan on medium-high heat. Cook artichoke in batches, for 2 to 3 minutes each side or until charred and heated through. Transfer to a large heatproof bowl.

STEP 3

Add beans, pine nuts and rocket to warm artichoke. Place lemon juice and reserved marinade in a screw-top jar. Season with salt and pepper. Secure lid. Shake well. Pour over salad. Add parsley. Toss gently to combine. Serve.

NUTRITION VALUE

604 KJ Energy, 7.2g fat, 0.7g saturated fat, 7.1g fiber, 6.6g protein, 11.7g carbs.

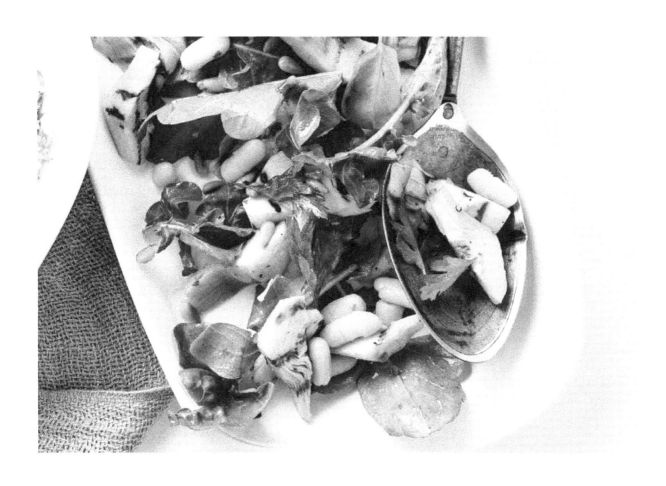

ASPARAGUS, AVOCADO AND CHERRY TOMATO SALAD

Add some crunch to the table with this healthy, gluten-free summer salad.

INGREDIENTS

60g baby spinach

250g cherry tomatoes, quartered

1 bunch mini asparagus, trimmed, halved lengthways

1/4 cup chopped walnuts, toasted

1 avocado, sliced

LEMON AND CHIVE DRESSING

2 tablespoons lemon juice

1 tablespoon olive oil

1 tablespoon finely chopped fresh chives

METHOD

STEP 1
Make Lemon and chive dressing: Place lemon juice, oil and chives in a screw-top jar. Season with salt and pepper. Secure lid. Shake until well combined.

STEP 2
Combine spinach, tomato, asparagus and walnuts in a bowl. Add avocado and dressing. Toss gently to combine. Serve.

NUTRITION VALUE	1005 KJ Energy, 23g fat, 4g saturated fat, 4g fiber, 4g protein, 3g carbs.

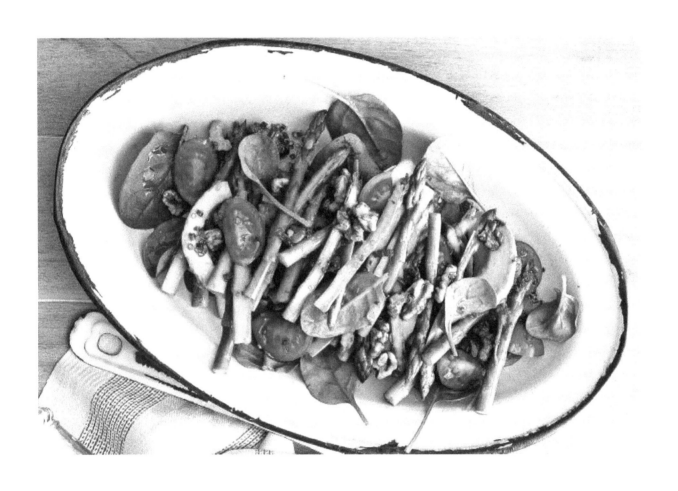

RAW PASTA PUTTANESCA

Marinated tomatoes, raw olives and herbs add zing to this raw puttanesca.

MAKES 4 SERVING/ TOTAL TIME 5 MINUTE

INGREDIENTS

4 cups chopped tomatoes (6 truss tomatoes)

1/2 cup halved Loving Earth raw olives or kalamata olives, pitted

1/4 cup diced white onion

1/4 cup cold pressed olive oil, plus 1 tablespoon to serve

2 tablespoons capers plus 1 tablespoon caper brine

2 teaspoons oregano leaves

2 teaspoons thyme leaves

2 teaspoons small basil leaves

2 teaspoons curly parsley leaves, roughly chopped

1 teaspoon chili flakes

3 cloves crushed garlic

Himalayan pink salt and pepper to taste

4 large zucchinis

1/4 cup pine nuts

METHOD

STEP 1
Mix all ingredients except for the pine nuts and zucchinis in a big bowl until well combined. Cover and refrigerate for at least 4 hours to marinate.

STEP 2
In a separate bowl, use a vegetable peeler to peel 1 cm wide strips from the zucchinis, they should resemble fettuccini. Add marinated vegetables to zucchinis and gently.

STEP 3
Divide into 4 bowls. Top with pine nuts, and drizzle with extra-virgin olive oil, to serve.

NUTRITION VALUE

1190 KJ Energy, 8.7g fat, 1.9g saturated fat, 13.6g fiber, 11.3g protein, 32.2g carbs.

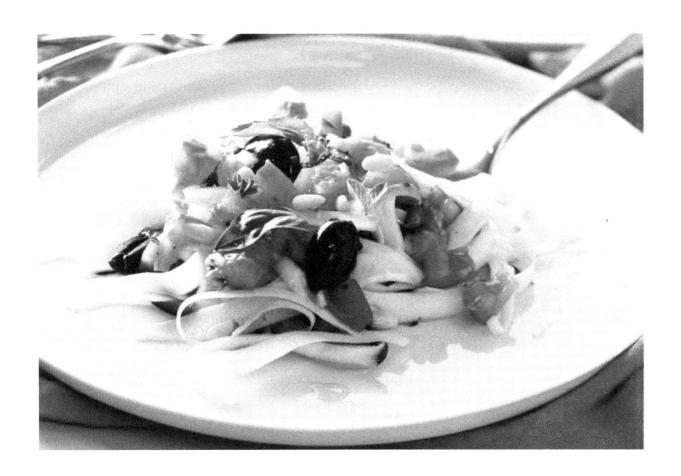

RAWKIN SUSHI ROLLS

Food process raw cauliflower and pine nuts to create a rice-like filling for these **gluten-free**, raw sushi rolls

MAKES 6 SERVING/ TOTAL TIME 35 MINUTE

INGREDIENTS

CAULIFLOWER SUSHI RICE

Half a head of cauliflower

1/2 cup pine nuts

1/2 cup sunflower seeds

2 tablespoons brown rice vinegar

Stevia, to taste

NORI ROLL

10 Nori Sheets

2 carrots, julienned

2 cucumbers, cut in half and sliced into 1cm sticks

2 large firm avocados, cut into 1 cm sticks

2 cups sprouts

DIPPING SAUCE

1/2 cup tamari

1 inch ginger, grated

2 tablespoons brown rice vinegar

METHOD

STEP 1

Pulse the cauliflower, pine nuts and sunflower seeds in a food processor.

STEP 2

Place one nori sheet onto a sushi mat shiny side down. Spoon a thin layer of the cauliflower "rice" along the nori sheet about 2 cm from the bottom edge the "rice" should cover about half the sheet and run all the way from the left edge of the nori sheet to the right edge.

Step 3

Place a 1-2 cm line of julienned carrots in the middle of the "rice" bed, running all the way across the nori sheet. Do the same with the cucumber and the avocado.

STEP 4

Using the sushi mat, carefully fold the bottom edge of the nori sheet over your row of vegies.

STEP 5

Using a sharp knife, gently slice the nori rolls into 2.5 cm pieces. Arrange on a serving platter.

STEP 6

Combine all the ingredients for the dipping sauce

NUTRITION VALUE	1632 KJ Energy, 35g fat, 6g saturated fat, 8g fiber, 9g protein, 7g carbs.

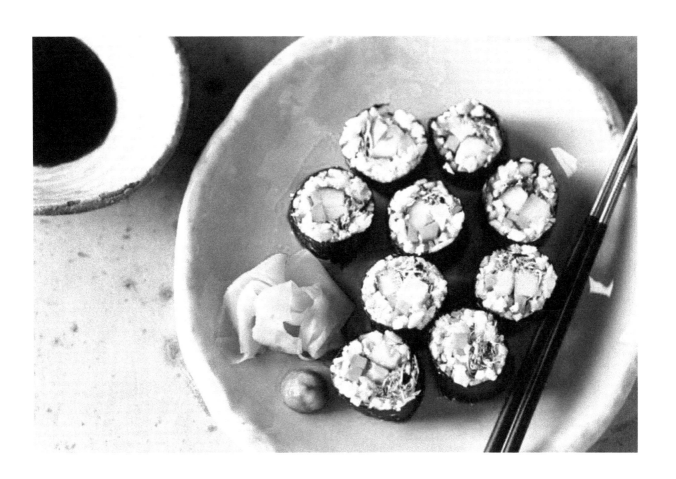

EASY GREEN SUPERFOOD SALAD

Sprouts and a tangy dressing give this lean, green salad texture and bite. Cubes of creamy avocado make it a meal.

MAKES 10 SERVING/ TOTAL TIME 10 MINUTE

INGREDIENTS

SALAD

4 cups mixed green salad leaves, tightly packed

2 cups sprout such as broccoli, sunflower, snow pea or alfalfa

2 medium cucumbers, chopped

1 avocado, cubed

1 tablespoon chia seeds

1 tablespoon sunflower seeds

1 tablespoon pumpkin seeds

Fresh curly parsley, to serve

DRESSING

1 tablespoon lemon juice

1/8 cup raw apple cider vinegar

1/4 cup cold pressed olive oil

1/2 heaped tablespoons wholegrain mustard

METHOD

STEP 1

Place all ingredients for the salad in a large salad bowl and toss until combined.

STEP 2

In a medium screw-top jar, shake up ingredients for the dressing until smooth. Pour over salad, toss thoroughly and top with fresh parsley to serve.

NUTRITION VALUE

1190 KJ Energy, 8.7g fat, 1.9g saturated fat, 13.6g fiber, 11.3g protein, 32.2g carbs.

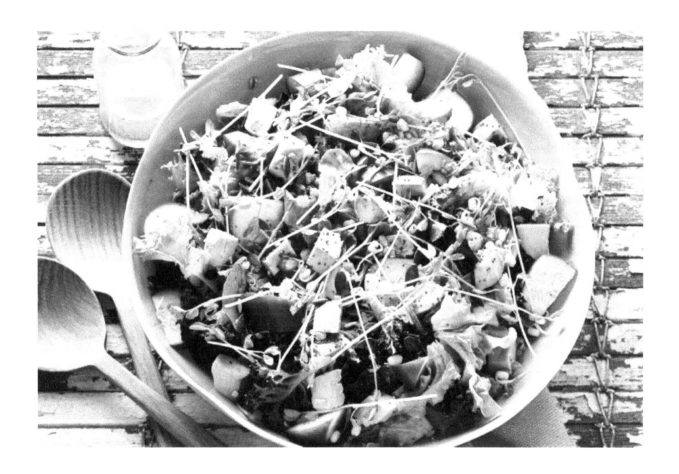

BARBECUED GARLIC AND HERB MUSHROOMS

Barbecues are not just meant for meats - grill up this fabulous mushroom side with garlic, thyme and rosemary.

MAKES 4 SERVING/ TOTAL TIME 10 MINUTE

INGREDIENTS

2 tablespoons extra-virgin Olive oil

2 garlic cloves, crushed

1 teaspoon finely chopped fresh thyme leaves

1 teaspoon finely chopped fresh rosemary leaves

4 (150g each) large flat mushrooms

Lemon wedges, to serve

METHOD

STEP 1

Preheat a barbecue chargrill on medium-high heat. Combine oil, garlic, thyme and rosemary in a bowl. Season with salt and pepper. Brush mushrooms with oil mixture.

STEP 2

Barbecue mushrooms for 6 to 8 minutes, turning halfway during cooking, or until charred and just tender. Transfer to a plate. Serve with lemon.

NUTRITION VALUE

511 KJ Energy, 8.9g fat, 1.2g saturated fat, 4.4g fiber, 5.6g protein, 2.7g carbs.

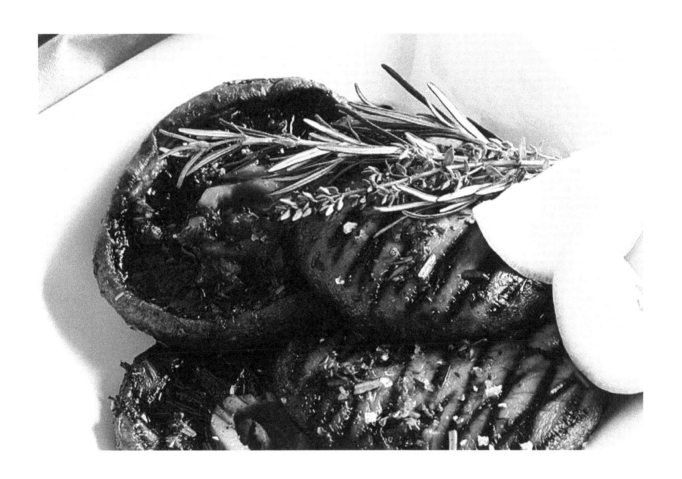

LENTIL AND ROAST CAPSICUM TABOULI

Make the most of ingredients at hand with this clever, quick solution side.

MAKES 4 SERVING/ TOTAL TIME 25 MINUTE

INGREDIENTS

1/2 cup burghul

1/3 cup boiling water

270g chargrilled capsicum, drained, finely chopped

1 cup fresh flat-leaf parsley leaves, finely chopped

1/3 cup fresh mint leaves, finely chopped

400g can lentils, drained, rinsed

1 teaspoon finely grated lemon rind

2 tablespoons lemon juice

1/2 teaspoon dried chili flakes (see note)

1 tablespoon olive oil

Lemon slices, to serve

Fresh parsley leaves, to serve

METHOD

STEP 1

Combine burghul and boiling water in a large heatproof bowl. Cover. Stand for 15 minutes or until water has absorbed.

STEP 2

Add capsicum, parsley, mint, lentils, lemon rind, lemon juice, chili and oil. Season with salt and pepper. Toss to combine. Top with lemon slices and parsley. Serve.

NUTRITION VALUE

931 KJ Energy, 6.6g fat, 1g saturated fat, 9.6g fiber, 8.5g protein, 25.9g carbs.

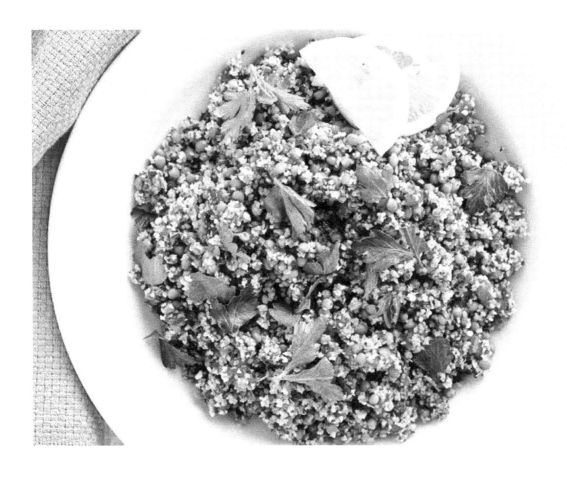

LENTIL, BARLEY AND MUSHROOM SOUP

Fast and fantastic vegetarian meals, using six ingredients!

MAKES 4 SERVING/ TOTAL TIME 50 MINUTE

INGREDIENTS

2 tablespoons olive oil

2 medium leeks, trimmed, halved, washed, thinly sliced

250g button mushrooms thinly sliced

2 x 410g cans chopped tomatoes (with basil and garlic)

3/4 cup red lentils

1/3 cup pearl barley

METHOD

STEP 1

Heat oil in a large saucepan over medium-high heat. Add leek and mushroom. Cook, stirring, for 3 to 4 minutes or until softened.

STEP 2

Add tomato, lentils, barley and 5 cups cold water. Season with salt and pepper. Cover. Bring to the boil. Reduce heat to low. Simmer for 35 to 40 minutes or until barley is tender. Ladle into bowls. Serve.

NUTRITION VALUE

1425 KJ Energy, 11g fat, 2g saturated fat, 12g fiber, 15g protein, 39g carbs.

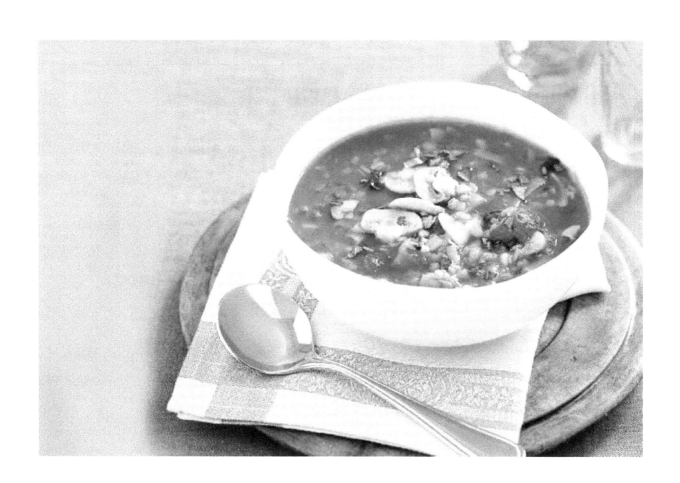

SPINACH & CELERIAC SALAD WITH WALNUTS

This delicious **vegan** side salad is a crunchy addition to the dinner table.

INGREDIENTS

100g pkt walnuts

60ml (1/4 cup) white wine vinegar

1 tablespoon olive oil

1 1/2 tablespoons brown sugar

2 tablespoons fresh lemon juice

1 celeriac, trimmed, peeled

1 bunch radish, trimmed, thinly sliced

140g pkt spinach, rocket & kale salad mix

METHOD

STEP 1

Heat a frying pan over medium heat. Cook the walnuts for 2-3 minutes or until lightly toasted. Set aside to cool.

STEP 2

Whisk the vinegar, oil and sugar in a jug until well combined. Season with salt and pepper.

STEP 3

Fill a large bowl with iced water. Add the lemon juice. Thinly slice the celeriac and place in the water. Place the radish in a large serving bowl.

STEP 4

Drain the celeriac. Add the walnuts, celeriac and salad mix to the radish. Add the dressing to the salad and toss to combine.

NUTRITION VALUE	755KJ Energy, 15g fat, 1 g saturated fat, 4g fiber, 4g protein, 7.5g carbs.

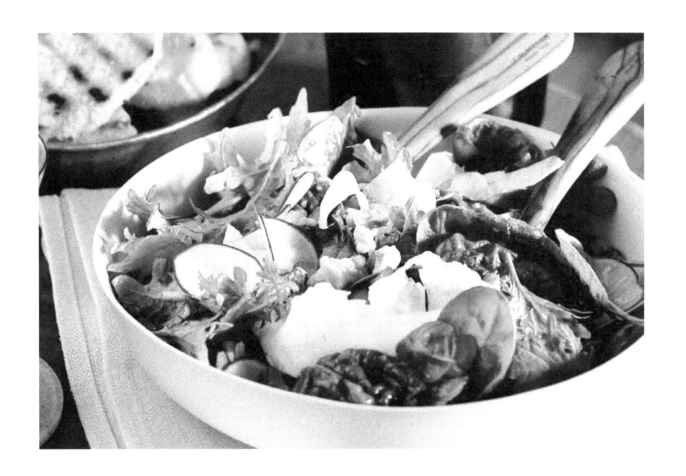

CANNELLINI BEAN AND LEMON SALAD

Gather around the table for a wonderful Italian banquet to share with friends and family.

MAKES 8 SERVING/ TOTAL TIME 10 MINUTE

INGREDIENTS

2 x 400g cans cannellini beans, drained, rinsed

400g can chickpeas, drained, rinsed

400g can lentils drained, rinsed

1/2 cup chopped fresh flat-leaf parsley leaves

1 tablespoon finely chopped fresh chives

DRESSING

2 teaspoons finely grated lemon rind

1 tablespoon lemon juice

2 tablespoons olive oil

1 small garlic clove, crushed

METHOD

STEP 1
Combine beans, chickpeas, lentils, parsley and chives in a bowl.

STEP 2
Make dressing Place lemon rind, lemon juice, oil and garlic in a screw-top jar. Season with salt and pepper. Secure lid. Shake to combine.

STEP 3
Toss dressing through salad. Serve.

NUTRITION VALUE	617 KJ Energy, 5.7g fat, 0.8g saturated fat, 6.8g fiber, 6.9g protein, 16g carbs.

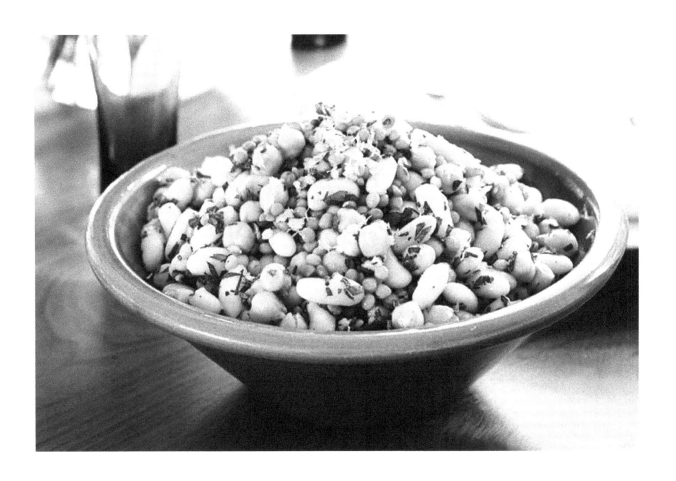

WILD RICE AND ROCKET SALAD

There's much to entice about this side with rice, it's delicious and low in price!

INGREDIENTS

1 cup Sunrise wild rice blend (with mushrooms)

1/2 red onion, halved, thinly sliced

1/2 cup semi-dried tomatoes, drained, halved

3/4 cup pitted kalamata olives

100g baby rocket

2 tablespoons red wine vinegar

2 tablespoons Bertolli extra-virgin olive oil

1 garlic clove, crushed

METHOD

STEP 1

Place rice and 2 cups cold water in a saucepan over high heat. Cover and bring to the boil. Reduce heat to low. Cook, covered, for 12 to 14 minutes or until liquid is absorbed. Set aside for 10 minutes to cool. Using a fork, stir rice to separate grains.

STEP 2

Combine rice, onion, tomato, olives and rocket in a bowl. Place vinegar, oil and garlic in a screw-top jar. Season with salt and pepper. Secure lid. Shake to combine.

STEP 3

Pour vinegar mixture over rice mixture. Toss to combine. Serve.

NUTRITION VALUE	1373 KJ Energy, 13g fat, 2g saturated fat, 7g fiber, 9g protein, 39g carbs.

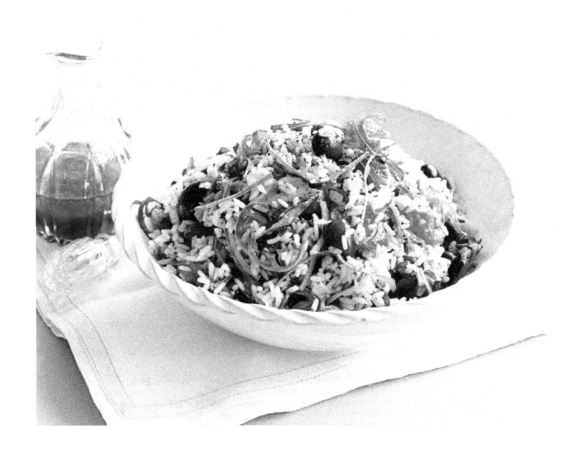

SICILIAN-STYLE STUFFED WHITE ZUCCHINIS

This pale green variety is sweet, mild and made for Mediterranean flavors.

MAKES 4 SERVING/ TOTAL TIME 30 MINUTE

INGREDIENTS

8 white zucchinis

70g (1/3 cup) couscous

50g (1/4 cup) raisins

1/2 teaspoon ground cinnamon

2 tablespoons tomato paste

1 garlic clove, finely chopped

Shredded fresh mint, to serve

METHOD

STEP 1

Use an apple corer, or a small sharp knife and a teaspoon, to remove the flesh from the center of the zucchinis, leaving a 5mm-thick border.

STEP 2

Place the couscous, raisins and cinnamon in a bowl. Season with salt and pepper. Stir until well combined.

STEP 3

Fill each zucchinis shell about three-quarters full with the couscous mixture. Place the zucchinis, in a single layer, in a large saucepan. Cover with cold water. Add the tomato paste, garlic, salt and pepper. Gently stir the sauce, being careful not to disturb the zucchinis. Bring to the boil over high heat. Reduce heat to low. Cook for 1 hour or until the zucchinis is tender.

STEP 4

Transfer zucchinis to a serving dish. Cut in half lengthways.

NUTRITION VALUE	610 KJ Energy, 1g fat, 6g fiber, 8 protein, 25g carbs.

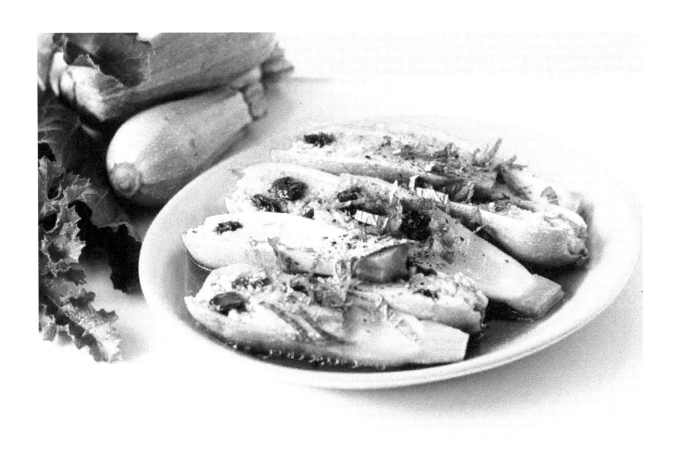

MISO BROTH WITH SILKEN TOFU AND ASIAN GREENS

Vegetarian cooking has never been easier with this speedy tofu soup.

MAKES 4 SERVING/ TOTAL TIME 15 MINUTE

INGREDIENTS

1L (4 cups) Massel vegetable liquid stock

1 tablespoon brown miso paste*

1 bunch baby bok choy

1 bunch choy sum

200g silken tofu, cut into small cubes

1 pack enoki mushrooms*, trimmed

METHOD

STEP 1

Place the vegetable stock in a large saucepan over high heat and bring to the boil. Reduce the heat to low, then stir in the miso paste and whisk until well combined.

STEP 2

Add the bok choy and choy sum leaves, then remove the saucepan from the heat. Ladle the stock and greens into 4 serving bowls.

STEP 3

Top with the tofu and garnish with the enoki mushrooms.

NUTRITION VALUE

1190 KJ Energy, 8.7g fat, 1.9g saturated fat, 13.6g fiber, 11.3g protein, 32.2g carbs.

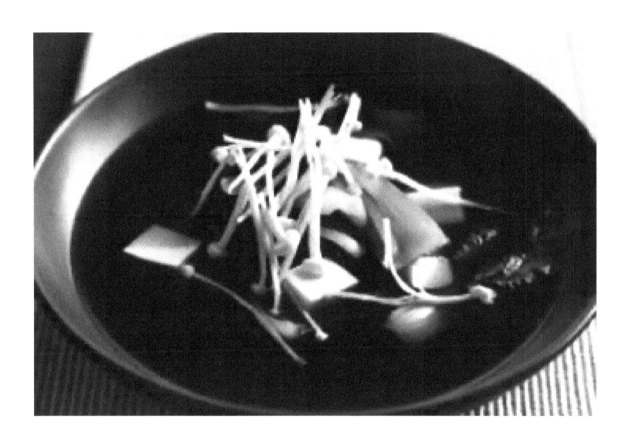

ASIAN GREENS WITH TOFU AND MUSHROOM

Mixed mushrooms and Asian greens star in this aromatic Asian side dish

MAKES 4 SERVING/ TOTAL TIME 25 MINUTE

INGREDIENTS

2 teaspoons sesame oil

2 garlic cloves, chopped finely

1 tablespoon ginger (cut into thin 4cm lengths)

1/2 cup (125ml) oyster sauce

1 tablespoon peanut oil

1 bunch baby bok choy, trimmed

1 bunch baby gai lan (Chinese broccoli), trimmed and cut into 15cm lengths

1 bunch choy sum, trimmed and cut into 15cm lengths

350g mixed Asian mushrooms, trimmed

1 packet silken firm tofu, drained, cut into 4cm cubes

Toasted sesame seeds, to serve

METHOD

STEP 1

Heat half the sesame oil in a wok or large, deep non-stick frying pan over medium-high heat. Add the garlic and ginger and cook for 30 seconds. Add the oyster sauce and cook for 30 seconds or until heated through. Remove from heat, cover and set aside until needed.

STEP 2

Wipe the wok clean. Heat the remaining sesame oil and peanut oil over medium-high heat. Add the bok choy, gai larn and choy sum and stir-fry for 3 minutes. Add the mushrooms and stir-fry for another 2 minutes.

STEP 3

Remove from heat and arrange on a serving plate. Top with the tofu and drizzle with the warm oyster sauce mixture. Sprinkle with sesame seeds and serve immediately. Serve with rice or noodles.

NUTRITION VALUE	1184 KJ Energy, 13g fat, 2g saturated fat, 19g fiber, 19g protein, 15g carbs.

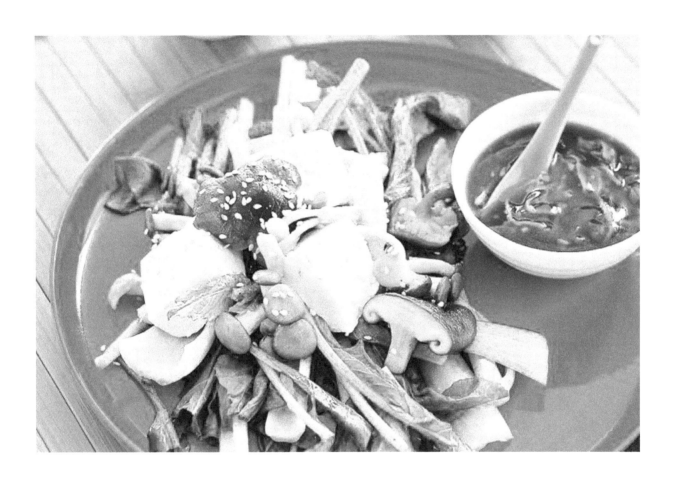

VEGETABLE RATATOUILLE

Make your own fresh and vibrant ratatouille for a wholesome vegetarian meal.

MAKES 4 SERVING/ TOTAL TIME 30 MINUTE

INGREDIENTS

2 teaspoons olive oil

3 zucchinis, ends trimmed, halved lengthways, thinly sliced

3 Lebanese eggplants, ends trimmed, halved lengthways, thinly sliced

1 red capsicum, halved, deseeded, finely chopped

1 brown onion, halved, thinly sliced

1 garlic clove, crushed

2 x 400g cans chopped tomatoes

2 tablespoons tomato paste

100g green beans, topped, coarsely chopped

1/4 cup finely shredded fresh basil

Creamy polenta, to serve

METHOD

STEP 1
Heat the oil in a large, deep frying pan over medium heat. Add the zucchinis, eggplant, capsicum, onion and garlic and cook, stirring, for 3 minutes or until onion softens.

STEP 2
Reduce heat to low. Add the tomato and tomato paste and cook, uncovered, stirring occasionally, for 15 minutes or until mixture thickens slightly.

STEP 3
Add the beans and cook for 5 minutes or until beans are bright green and tender crisp. Remove from heat and stir through the basil.

STEP 4
Divide the lemon & thyme polenta among serving plates. Top with the vegetable ratatouille and serve immediately.

NUTRITION VALUE

100 KJ Energy, 3g fat, 0.5g saturated fat, 6g fiber, 4g protein, 10g carbs.

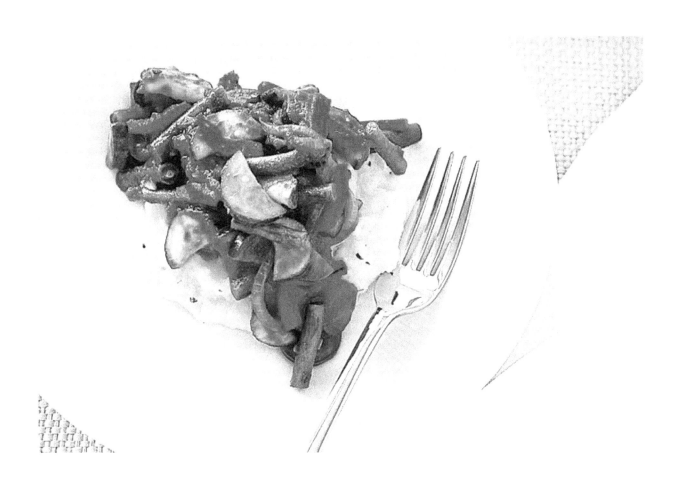

ITALIAN VEGETABLE SALAD

This Italian salad is a beautiful combination of flavors, colors and textures.

MAKES 8 SERVING/ TOTAL TIME 40 MINUTE

INGREDIENTS

2 tablespoons olive oil

3 red onions, cut into wedges

2 red capsicums, deseeded, thickly sliced

175g baby beans, topped

500g grape tomatoes, halved

300g marinated artichokes, drained, halved

150g small black olives, drained

2 teaspoons balsamic vinegar

METHOD

STEP 1

Preheat oven to 220°C. Combine oil, onions and capsicums in a roasting pan. Roast for 30 minutes, turning once, or until edges are crisp. Cool to room temperature.

STEP 2

Cook beans in a saucepan of boiling water for 2 minutes or until just tender. Drain. Rinse under cold water. Pat dry.

STEP 3

Combine all ingredients, and salt and pepper in a large bowl. Toss gently. Serve.

NUTRITION VALUE	523 KJ Energy, 9g fat, 1g saturated fat, 3g protein, 5g carbs.

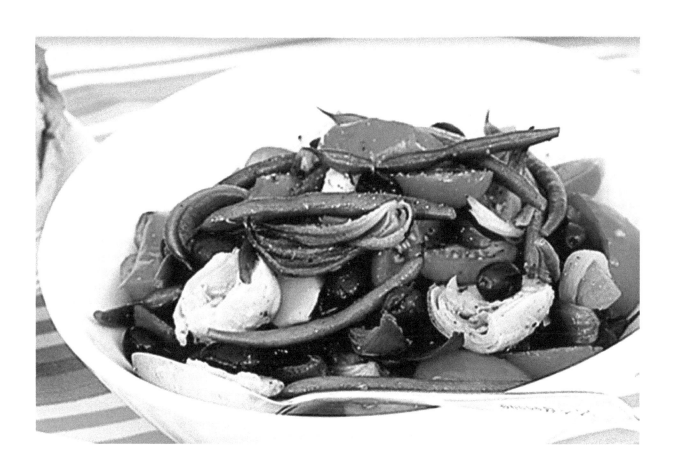

ASPARAGUS WITH SESAME DRESSING

Asian sesame seed dressing is delicious when served with fresh green asparagus.

MAKES 6 SERVING/ TOTAL TIME 10 MINUTE

INGREDIENTS

3 bunches asparagus

2 tablespoons white sesame seed paste

2 tablespoons caster sugar

1/3 cup (80ml) cooking sake

2 tablespoons soy sauce

2 tablespoons sesame seeds

METHOD

STEP 1

Trim ends from asparagus, then using a sharp knife, cut on a severe angle so that each slice is about 10cm long. Cook asparagus in a large saucepan of boiling salted water for 30-60 seconds or until almost tender. Refresh under cold running water, then drain. Pat dry with paper towel.

STEP 2

Combine sesame paste, sugar, sake and soy sauce in a large bowl. Add asparagus and toss to coat in dressing. Serve sprinkled with sesame seeds

NUTRITION VALUE

1190 KJ Energy, 8.7g fat, 1.9g saturated fat, 13.6g fiber, 11.3g protein, 32.2g carbs.

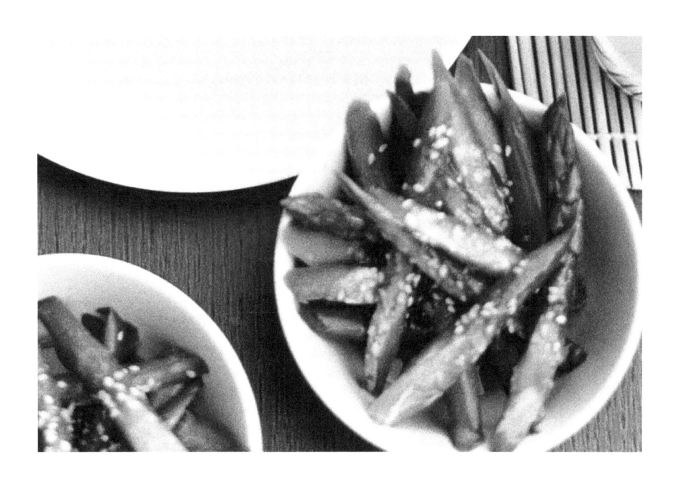

PINK GRAPEFRUIT & CUCUMBER SALAD

Balsamic vinegar cuts through the flavors of the grapefruit and cucumber in this summer salad with a difference.

INGREDIENTS

1 large pink grapefruit, peeled, white pith removed

100g mixed salad leaves

1 Lebanese cucumber, halved, thinly sliced

60g snow peas, trimmed, thinly sliced lengthways

1 1/2 tablespoons balsamic vinegar

METHOD

STEP 1
Use a small sharp knife to remove the grapefruit segments, cutting close to either side of the white membrane. Discard membrane.

STEP 2
Place the grapefruit, salad leaves, cucumber and snow peas in a bowl and toss to combine. Divide among serving bowls. Drizzle over the balsamic vinegar and serve.

NUTRITION VALUE

135KJ Energy, 0.5g fat,
2g fiber, 2g protein, 5g carbs.

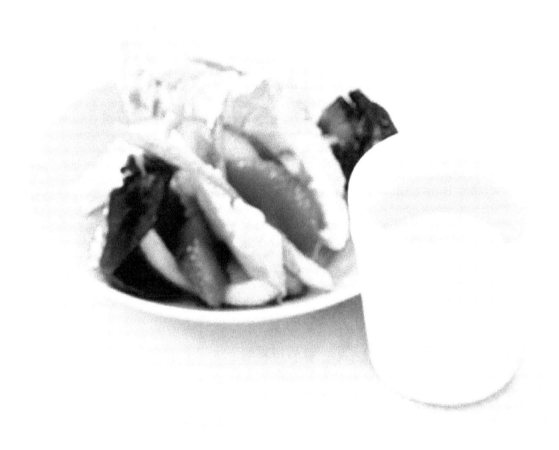

CUCUMBER, RADISH AND SNOW PEA SALAD

For the perfect accompaniment to a summer meal, whip up this crunchy salad.

MAKES 8 SERVING/ TOTAL TIME 10 MINUTE

INGREDIENTS

4 Lebanese cucumbers

1 bunch radishes, washed, trimmed

1 cup mint leaves

150g snow peas, thinly sliced diagonally

50g snow pea sprouts, trimmed

1/4 cup lime juice

1 tablespoon olive oil

METHOD

STEP 1

Using a vegetable peeler, peel cucumbers lengthways to form long thin ribbons. Discard excess seeds. Place cucumber ribbons into a bowl. Thinly slice radishes into rounds. Cut into thin strips. Add to cucumber with mint, snow peas and sprouts. Cover. Refrigerate until required.

STEP 2

Combine lime juice, oil, and salt and pepper in a jug. Whisk to combine. Add dressing to salad just before serving. Toss until well combined. Serve.

NUTRITION VALUE

191 KJ Energy, 2.5g fat, 0.3g saturated fat, 1.9 fiber, 1.7g protein, 3.9g carbs.

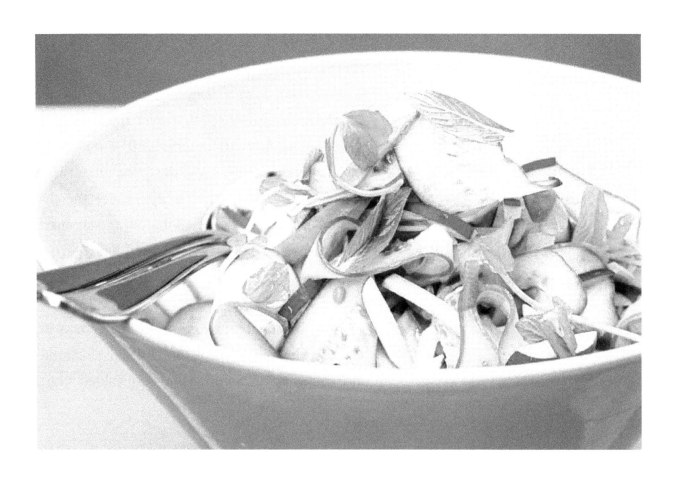

FOUR-BEAN SOUP WITH BARLEY

This hearty bean soup is filling enough to be a main course all on its own.

MAKES 4 SERVING/ TOTAL TIME 50 MINUTE

INGREDIENTS

1 tablespoon olive oil

1 onion, roughly chopped

3 garlic cloves, sliced

1 celery stalk, roughly chopped

1 carrot, roughly chopped

3 thyme sprigs

1/2 cup (105g) pearl barley

2 cups (500ml) Massel vegetable liquid stock

2 x 400g cans four-bean mix, rinsed, drained

400g can chopped tomatoes

1/2 cup finely sliced flat-leaf parsley leaves

METHOD

STEP 1

Heat the oil in a large, deep saucepan over low heat. Add the onion, garlic, celery, carrot and thyme, and cook, stirring, for 8-10 minutes until onion is soft. Add the barley and stir to coat in the onion mixture. Add the vegetable stock and 1 liter (4 cups) water, then bring to the boil. Reduce heat to medium-low and simmer for 20 minutes or until barley is slightly tender.
Pause

STEP 2

Add the beans and tomato, and stir to combine. Bring back to a simmer and cook for a further 15 minutes or until barley is soft. Serve in bowls sprinkled with parsley.

NUTRITION VALUE	1232 KJ Energy, 6.3g fat, 1.1g saturated fat, 14.6g fiber, 12g protein, 41.3g carbs.

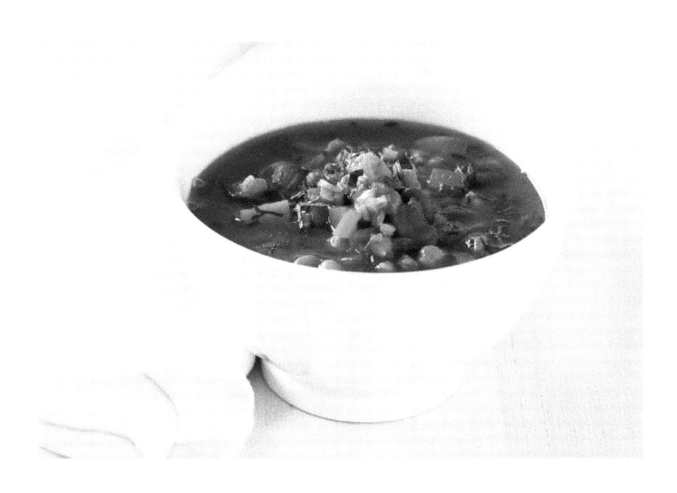

HEARTY VEGETABLE SOUP WITH CHICKPEAS

Get your five serves of veggies a day, the easy way in this hearty soup.

MAKES 4 SERVING/ TOTAL TIME 80 MINUTE

INGREDIENTS

2 teaspoons olive oil

1 large brown onion, chopped

2 teaspoons ground turmeric

1 teaspoon ground coriander

2 teaspoons ground cumin

5 cups chopped vegetables

3 cups Massel vegetable liquid stock

2 cups water

415g can chopped tomatoes

400g can chickpeas, drained, rinsed

1/2 cup flat-leaf parsley, chopped

METHOD

STEP 1

Heat oil in a large saucepan over medium-high heat. Add onion. Cook for 3 minutes. Add spices and firm vegetables (such as pumpkin, potatoes, carrots, capsicum and celery). Stir to coat.

STEP 2

Stir in stock, water, tomatoes and chickpeas. Bring to the boil. Reduce heat to medium-low. Simmer, uncovered, for 40 minutes or until vegetables are soft. Add tender vegetables (such as beans, broccoli, peas, zucchinis). Cook for a further 5 minutes. Stir in parsley. Season with pepper. Serve.

NUTRITION VALUE

1135 KJ Energy, 11.9g fat, 1.8g saturated fat, 9.5g fiber, 9.5g protein, 27.4g carbs.

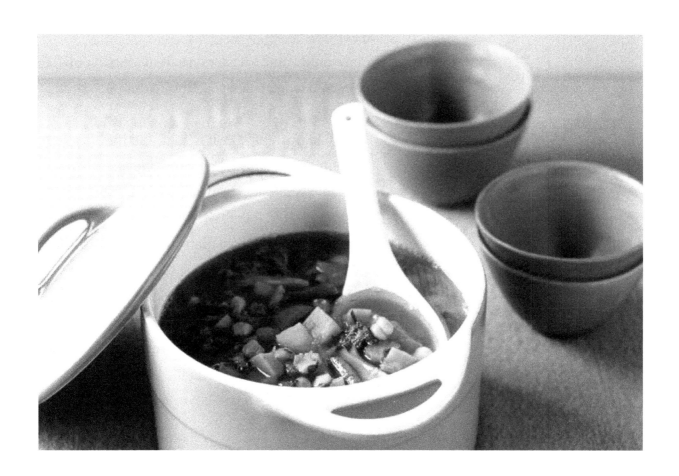

PANZANELLA

With this Italian bread salad, you'll give pizza and pasta a run come summer.

MAKES 6 SERVING/ TOTAL TIME 50 MINUTE

INGREDIENTS

1/2 red onion, thinly sliced

2 small red capsicums, quartered, seeded

1/2 (330g) loaf day-old ciabatta, cut into 3cm pieces

100ml extra-virgin olive oil, plus extra, to drizzle

1 clove garlic, crushed

3 anchovy fillets, finely chopped

1 long red chili, seeded, finely chopped

60ml (1/4 cup) red wine vinegar

200g grape tomatoes

2 tablespoons baby capers

50g small black olives

5 vine-ripened tomatoes, cut into wedges

2 Lebanese cucumbers, halved, cut into 2cm pieces

1/4 cup small basil leaves

METHOD

STEP 1

Place onion and 1 teaspoon salt in a small bowl, cover with cold water, then soak for 20 minutes. Drain.

STEP 2

Meanwhile, preheat grill to high and line an oven tray with foil. Place capsicums, skin-side up, on tray and cook for 15 minutes or until skin is blistered and blackened. Fold foil up over capsicums and cool for 10 minutes. Peel off skins, then cut into 5mm-thick strips.

STEP 3

Place bread on an oven tray, drizzle generously with extra oil, then season with salt and pepper. Cook under grill, turning frequently, for 10 minutes To make dressing, place garlic, anchovies, chili, vinegar and 1/2 teaspoon salt in a small bowl. Whisk to combine, then gradually whisk in oil.

STEP 5

Using your hands, squeeze each grape tomato, bursting skin and squirting juice over bread, then add tomatoes to bowl ,Divide among plates to serve.

NUTRITION VALUE

1448 KJ Energy, 19g fat, 3g saturated fat, 9g protein, 33g carbs.

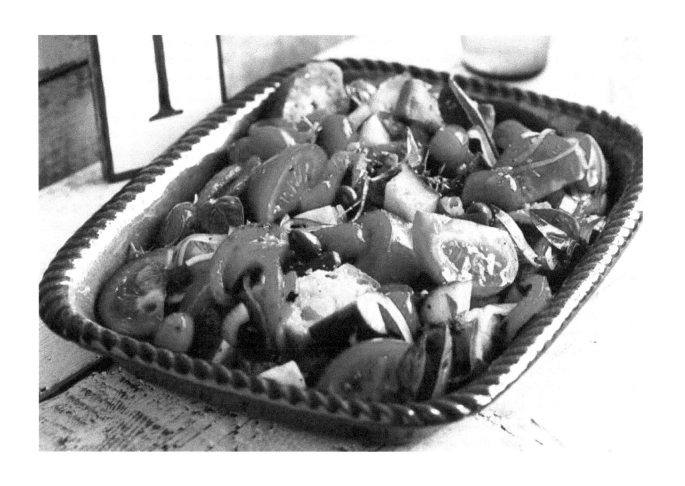

ROAST VEGETABLE SALAD

This recipe is **vegan** friendly.

MAKES 4 SERVING/ TOTAL TIME 60 MINUTE

INGREDIENTS

1 small kumara (orange sweet potato), chopped

160g pumpkin, chopped

2 small Desiree potatoes, peeled and chopped

1 medium carrot, peeled and sliced

2 small onions, sliced

2 cloves garlic, crushed

1 tablespoon chopped fresh rosemary

1 tablespoon olive oil

420g can Edgell Four Bean Mix, drained

1 tablespoon balsamic vinegar

rosemary, to garnish

crusty toasted bread, to serve

METHOD

STEP 1

Preheat oven to 200°C. Line a large baking tray with non-stick baking paper.

STEP 2

Combine kumara, pumpkin, potatoes, carrot, onions, garlic, rosemary and oil in a large bowl. Mix until vegetables are evenly coated with oil. Season with salt and pepper.

STEP 3

Place vegetables in a single layer in a large baking dish. Roast for 35 minutes.

STEP 4

Place vegetables into a large bowl and stir in beans and vinegar. Garnish with rosemary. Serve with toasted bread.

NUTRITION VALUE

777 KJ Energy, 5g fat, 1g saturated fat, 8g fiber, 8g protein, 23g carbs.

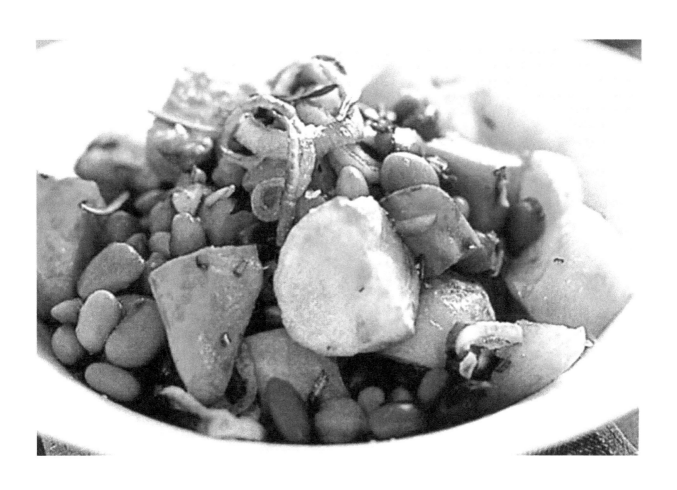

MUSHROOM & ASPARAGUS SALAD WITH VINAIGRETTE

This recipe is **vegan** friendly.

MAKES 4 SERVING/ TOTAL TIME 40 MINUTE

INGREDIENTS

500g flat mushrooms quartered

200g Swiss brown mushrooms, ends trimmed

150g oyster mushrooms, halved

Olive oil spray

2 bunches asparagus, woody ends trimmed, halved lengthways

1 1/2 tablespoons red wine vinegar

1 tablespoon olive oil

1 garlic clove, crushed

1/2 teaspoon caster sugar

1 small red onion, cut into thin wedges

100g baby rocket leaves

2 tablespoons chopped fresh chives

METHOD

STEP1

Preheat oven to 160°C. Line a baking tray with non-stick baking paper. Arrange the combined mushroom, in a single layer, on the lined tray. Lightly spray with olive oil spray and season with salt and pepper. Bake in oven for 20 minutes or until the mushroom is tender.

STEP 2

Meanwhile, cook the asparagus in a medium saucepan of boiling water until bright green and tender crisp. Refresh under cold running water. Drain. Whisk together the vinegar, oil, garlic and sugar in a small bowl.

STEP 3

Place the asparagus, onion and rocket in a large bowl. Add the mushroom and vinegar mixture and gently toss until just combined. Taste and season with pepper. Divide the salad among serving bowls and sprinkle with chives. Serve immediately.

NUTRITION VALUE	465 KJ Energy, 5g fat, 1g saturated fat, 6g fiber, 10g protein, 3g carbs.

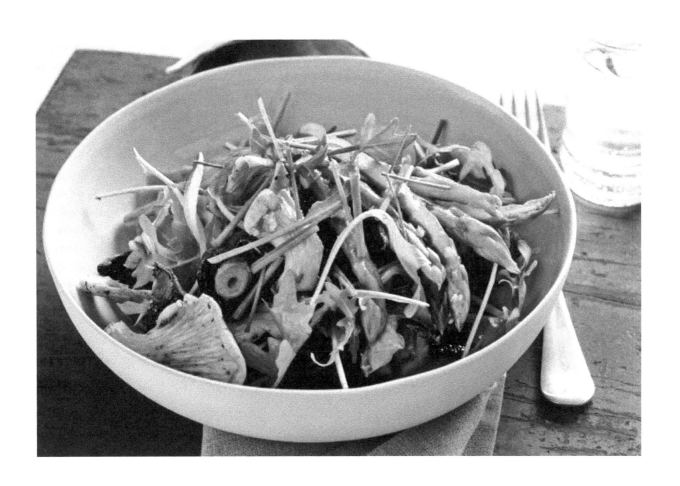

ROAST BEETROOT & WALNUT SALAD

Try a salad with a difference with this roasted beetroot and walnut version.

MAKES 6 SERVING/ TOTAL TIME 70 MINUTE

INGREDIENTS

8 medium beetroot, ends trimmed

100g walnut kernels

1 red onion, finely chopped

60ml (1/4 cup) red wine vinegar

60ml (1/4 cup) extra-virgin olive oil

1 teaspoon ground cumin

1 orange

1/2 cup chopped fresh continental parsley

METHOD

STEP 1

Preheat oven to 200C. Wrap each beetroot bulb in foil. Place on a baking tray. Bake for 1 hour or until tender when pierced with a skewer. Set aside to cool slightly. Wearing rubber gloves to avoid staining your hands, peel the beetroot. Cut into 3cm pieces.

STEP 2

Meanwhile, heat a large frying pan over medium heat. Add the walnuts and cook, stirring often, for 1 minute or until aromatic.

STEP 3

Combine walnuts and onion in a large bowl. Whisk the vinegar, oil and cumin in a jug. Season with salt and pepper. Use a zester to remove the rind from orange. (Alternatively, use a vegetable peeler to peel the rind from orange. Use a small sharp knife to remove white pith from the rind. Cut the rind into very thin strips.)

STEP 4

Add beetroot and dressing to the walnut mixture. Gently toss to combine. Cover and set aside to develop the flavors.

NUTRITION VALUE

1180 KJ Energy, 21g fat, 2g saturated fat, 7.5g fiber, 6.5g protein, 17g carbs.

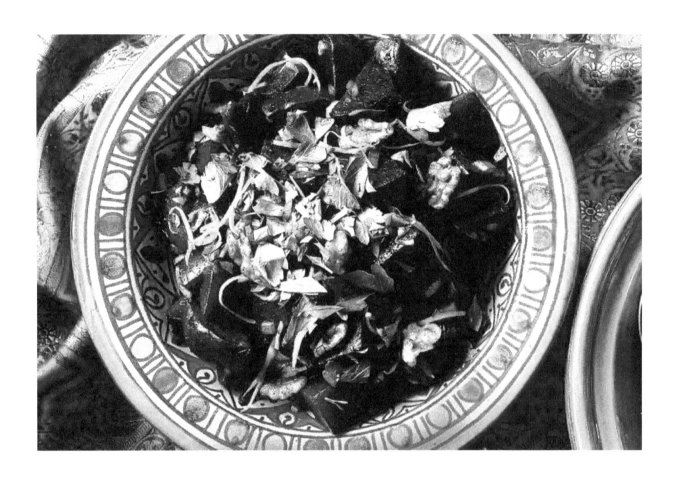

WATERCRESS AND FIG SALAD

Making a tasty salad with just five ingredients is easier than you think

INGREDIENTS

1/4 cup (45g) hazelnuts

1/3 cup (80ml) balsamic vinegar

2 cups watercress sprigs

2 ripe figs, broken into quarters

1 tablespoon hazelnut oil

METHOD

STEP 1

Preheat oven to 200°C. Place hazelnuts in a roasting pan and cook for 5 minutes or until toasted. Place hazelnuts in a clean tea towel and rub to remove skins (this is easiest when hazelnuts are still warm). Cut hazelnuts in half and set aside.

STEP 2

Meanwhile, place vinegar in a small saucepan over high heat. Bring to the boil. Reduce heat to medium-high and simmer for 5 minutes or until reduced to 1 1/2 tablespoons. Set aside to cool.

STEP 3

Arrange watercress sprigs, figs and hazelnuts on serving plates. Drizzle with balsamic reduction and hazelnut oil and serve immediately.

NUTRITION VALUE

1190 KJ Energy, 8.7g fat, 1.9g saturated fat, 13.6g fiber, 11.3g protein, 32.2g carbs.

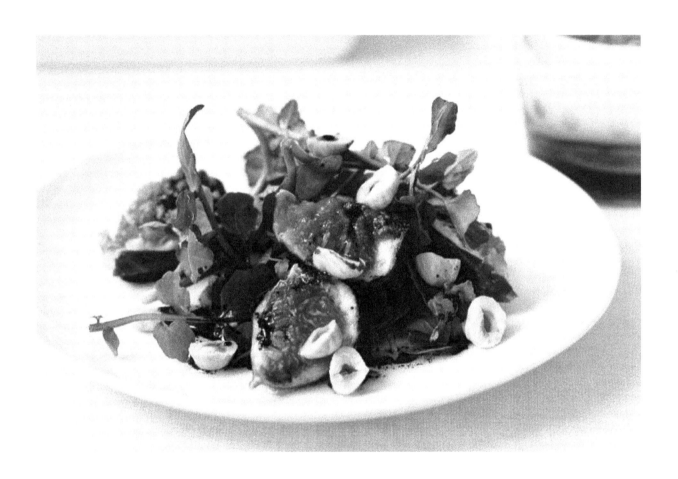

SUGAR SNAP PEA, ROASTED SHIITAKE & BLACK BEAN SALAD

Create something different with this gourmet Asian salad topped with roasted shiitake mushrooms.

MAKES 6 SERVING/ TOTAL TIME 20 MINUTE

INGREDIENTS

12 fresh shiitake mushrooms

250g snow pea sprouts, long ends trimmed

150g sugar snap peas, trimmed, blanched, refreshed

1 cup canned black beans, rinsed, drained (see Notes)

DRESSING

1/2 cup (125ml) vegetable oil

1 tablespoon sesame oil

1/4 cup (60ml) rice vinegar

1/4 cup (60ml) soy sauce

1 teaspoon hot chili sauce

1 tablespoon brown sugar

METHOD

STEP 1

Preheat the oven to 190°C.

STEP 2

Whisk dressing ingredients together.

STEP 3

Brush shiitakes with a little dressing, then place in a baking dish in the oven for 10 minutes, turning once. Cool.

STEP 4

Combine the sprouts, peas and beans with the remaining dressing. Serve the salad topped with roasted shiitakes.

NUTRITION VALUE

1476 KJ Energy, 23g fat, 3g saturated fat, 5g fiber, 10g protein, 23g carbs.

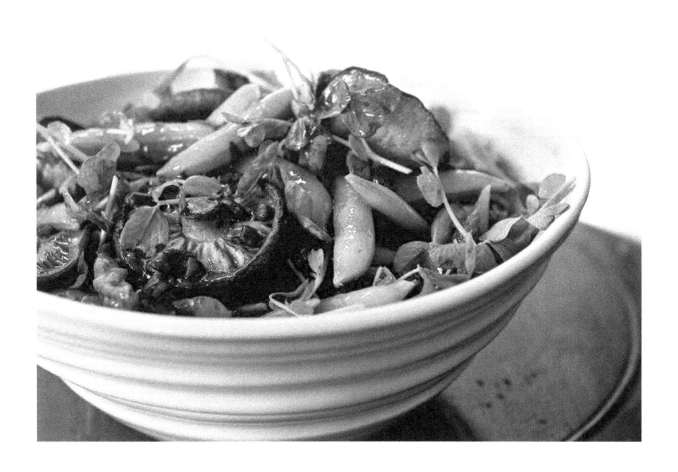

WITLOF SALAD

Even the kids could make this simple green salad.

MAKES 4 SERVING/ TOTAL TIME 10 MINUTE

INGREDIENTS

2 witlof, bases trimmed, leaves separated

1 x 100g pkt sweet baby greens with herbs

1 1/2 tablespoons olive oil

1 tablespoon balsamic vinegar

Salt & freshly ground black pepper

METHOD

STEP 1

Arrange witlof on a serving plate and top with baby greens.

STEP 2

Place the oil and vinegar in a screw-top jar and shake until well combined. Taste and season with salt and pepper. Drizzle salad with dressing and serve immediately.

NUTRITION VALUE

300 KJ Energy, 7.5g fat, 1g saturated fat, 1.5g fiber,0.5g protein, 1.5g carbs.

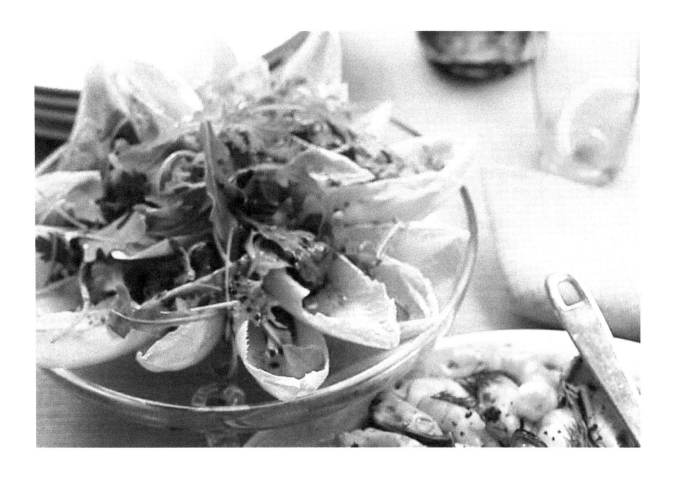

BITTER LEAF SALAD

Fennel, witlof and radicchio are combined in this healthy and unique gourmet salad.

INGREDIENTS

1/4 cup (60ml) extra-virgin olive oil

Juice of 1 lemon

2 cups wild rocket

1 bunch watercress, stalks trimmed

1 radicchio, outer leaves discarded, inner leaves torn

1 witlof*, leaves separated

1 baby fennel, very thinly sliced

METHOD

STEP 1
Whisk the oil and lemon juice in a bowl, and season with salt and pepper.

STEP 2
Place the remaining ingredients in a large serving bowl, pour over the dressing and gently toss to combine. Serve immediately.

NUTRITION VALUE

1190 KJ Energy, 8.7g fat, 1.9g saturated fat, 13.6g fiber, 11.3g protein, 32.2g carbs.

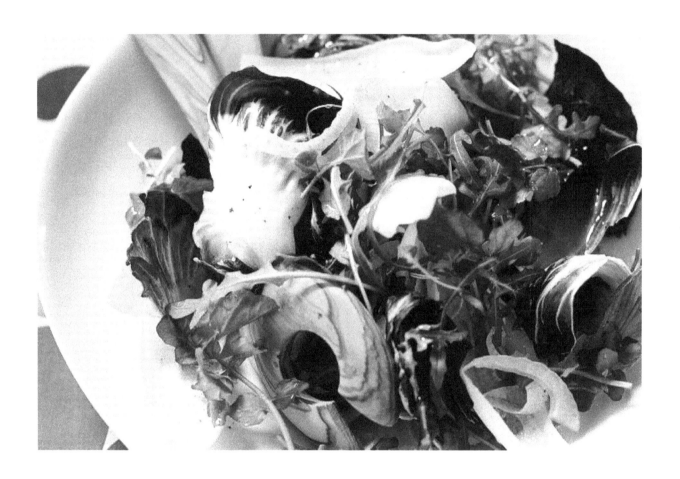

TOP-TO-TAIL CARROT SALAD

Use the whole carrot from top to tail in this hearty vegetarian side salad.

INGREDIENTS

3 bunches baby rainbow carrots, scrubbed or peeled, trimmed

2 tablespoons extra-virgin olive oil

Salt flakes, to season

1/2 bunch fresh tarragon

150g (2/3 cup) pearl barley, rinsed

CARROT TOP AND TARRAGON PISTOU

40g (2 cups) fresh carrot tops

2 tablespoons chopped fresh tarragon

45g (1/4 cup) pepitas, toasted

1 garlic clove, chopped

125ml (1/2 cup) extra-virgin olive oil

METHOD

STEP 1

Preheat the oven to 220C/200C fan forced. Place the carrots in a large roasting pan. Drizzle with oil, season with salt and toss to combine. Roast for 20 minutes. Add the tarragon and toss to combine. Roast for a further 20 minutes or until carrots are tender.

STEP 2

Meanwhile, cook the barley in a saucepan of boiling water for 35 minutes or until tender. Drain.

STEP 3

For the pistou, process all ingredients in a food processor until smooth.

STEP 4

Serve the carrots on a bed of barley, drizzled with the pistou. Season.

NUTRITION VALUE

1190 KJ Energy, 8.7g fat, 1.9g saturated fat, 13.6g fiber, 11.3g protein, 32.2g carbs.

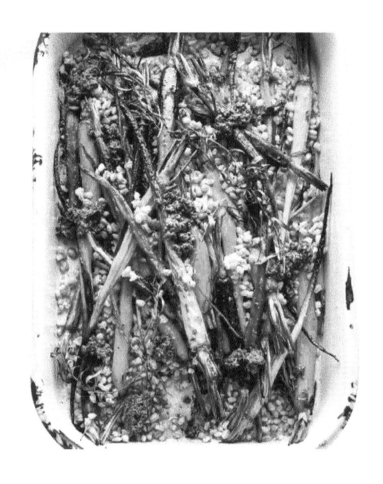

ROASTED VEGETABLE SALAD WITH FENNEL AND CHILIVINIAGRETTE

Roast veggies with a fennel and chili kicker - you'll forget it's a salad!

MAKES 4 SERVING/ TOTAL TIME 70 MINUTE

INGREDIENTS

3 baby sweet potatoes, halved lengthways

Olive oil cooking spray

1 eggplant, halved lengthways, sliced

200g grape tomatoes

120g packet spinach and beetroot salad leaves

2 spring onion bulbs, thinly sliced

2 tablespoons pepita and sunflower seed mix

FENNEL AND CHILIVINAIGRETTE

2 teaspoons fennel seeds

1 long red chili, seeded, finely chopped

1/4 cup extra-virgin olive oil

2 tablespoons apple cider vinegar

METHOD

STEP 1

Preheat oven to 220°C/200°C fan-forced. Line a large baking tray with baking paper.

STEP 2

Place sweet potato on tray. Spray with oil. Roast for 10 minutes. Add eggplant to tray. Spray with oil. Roast for a further 10 minutes. Add tomatoes to tray. Spray with oil. Season vegetables with salt and pepper. Roast for a further 10 to 15 minutes or until vegetables are golden and tender and tomatoes have collapsed. Set aside for 10 minutes to cool.

STEP 3

Meanwhile, make Fennel and Chili Vinaigrette Place fennel seeds, chili, oil and vinegar in a screw-top jar. Season with salt and pepper. Shake to combine.

STEP 4

Place leaves, roasted vegetables, tomatoes, onion and seed mix on a serving platter. Drizzle with dressing. Serve.

NUTRITION VALUE	1171 KJ Energy, 19.7g fat, 2.6g saturated fat, 7.1g fiber, 5.4g protein, 16.7g carbs.

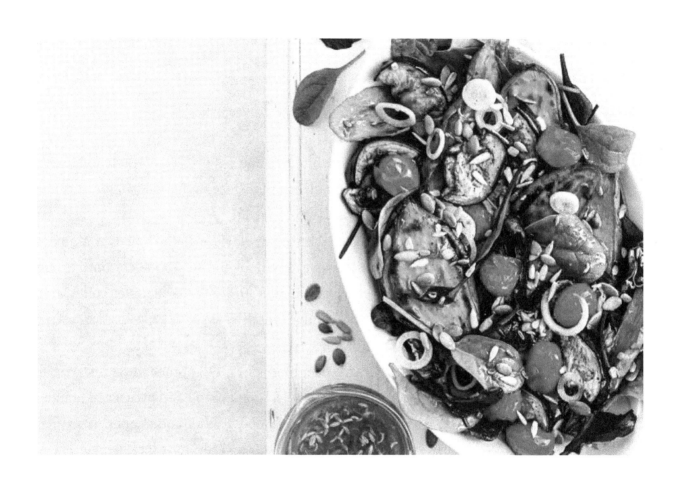

ASPARAGUS, LEMON AND PECAN WILD RICE SALAD

The colors of Christmas are reflected in this zingy wild rice salad. Crunchy pecans, fresh mint and pomegranate are the highlight flavors in this wonderful side dish.

MAKES 8 SERVING/ TOTAL TIME 55 MINUTE

INGREDIENTS

1 cup white long-grain rice

1/2 cup wild rice

2 bunches asparagus, trimmed

150g snow peas, trimmed

1 tablespoon lemon zest

1/4 cup fresh coriander leaves, chopped, plus extra leaves to serve

1/4 cup fresh mint leaves, chopped, plus extra leaves to serve

2 green onions, thinly sliced

2 tablespoons lemon juice

2 tablespoons extra-virgin olive oil

2 tablespoons preserved lemon, finely chopped

1/3 cup pecans, toasted, roughly chopped

150g tub pomegranate seeds

METHOD

STEP 1

Cook white rice and wild rice separately following packet directions. Rinse under cold water. Drain well.

STEP 2

Bring a saucepan of water to the boil over high heat. Add asparagus. Cook for 30 seconds or until bright green and tender. Drain. Refresh under cold water. Drain. Halve lengthways.

STEP 3

Place rice, snow peas, 1/2 of the lemon zest, coriander, mint, onion, lemon juice, oil and preserved lemon in a large bowl. Season with salt and pepper. Toss to combine. Transfer to a serving plate. Top with asparagus and sprinkle with pecans, pomegranate seeds, remaining lemon zest and extra coriander and mint leaves. Serve.

NUTRITION VALUE	1081 KJ Energy, 8.4g fat, 0.9g saturated fat, 3.3g fiber, 6g protein, 35.2g carbs.

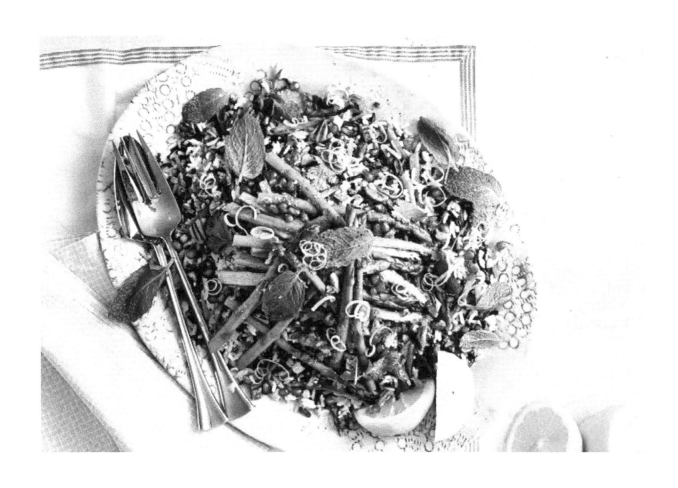

GRILLED ASPARAGUS AND TOMATO SALAD WITH PRESERVED LEMON

The combo of herbs with the preserved lemon dressing is the secret to this salad, adding loads of flavor, without extra fat.

MAKES 4 SERVING/ TOTAL TIME 25 MINUTE

INGREDIENTS

4 slices whole meal sourdough bread

2 bunches asparagus trimmed

1 1/2 tablespoons extra-virgin olive oil

1 garlic clove, peeled, halved

350g tomato medley, halved and quartered

200g grape tomatoes, whole and halved

1/2 cup fresh basil leaves

1/2 cup fresh continental parsley leaves

1 tablespoon baby salted capers, rinsed, drained, chopped

1 tablespoon white balsamic vinegar

1 preserved lemon quarters, pith removed, rinsed, finely chopped.

METHOD

STEP 1

Preheat a chargrill or barbecue grill plate on high. Brush the bread slices and asparagus with 1 tbs of the olive oil.

STEP 2

Grill the bread for 2 minutes each side or until lightly charred. Grill the asparagus for 1-2 minutes each side or until just tender. Transfer the bread and asparagus to a plate. Rub the bread with the cut side of the garlic clove and set aside to cool slightly.

STEP 3

Tear the bread into bite-size pieces. Combine the bread, asparagus, tomato, basil, parsley and capers in a large bowl. Season.

STEP 4

Whisk together the remaining olive oil, balsamic and preserved lemon. Add to the salad and gently toss to combine.

NUTRITION VALUE

648 KJ Energy, 1g fat, 8g saturated fat, 5g fiber, 6g protein, 13g carbs.

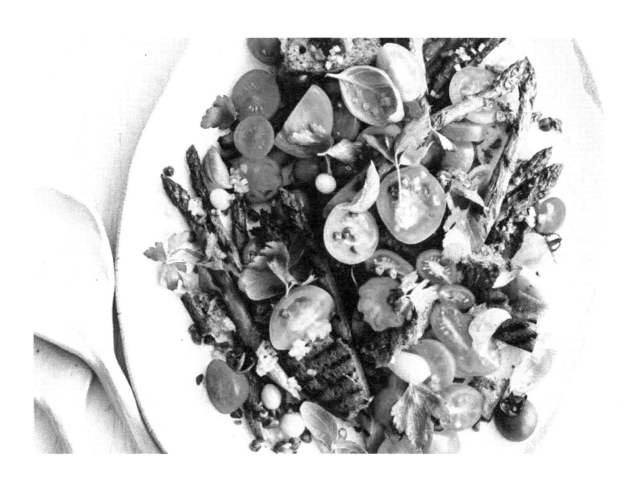

VEGETABLE TRAY BAKE WITH ROASTED GARLIC DRESSING

With high levels of vitamin C, garlic is good for you as well as for your food! Crushed, chopped or whole, this humble bulb adds deliciousness to simple sides.

MAKES 4 SERVING/ TOTAL TIME 55 MINUTE

INGREDIENTS

2 medium zucchinis, thickly sliced diagonally

400g butternut pumpkin peeled, cut into 3cm pieces

1 medium red capsicum, cut into 4cm pieces

1 medium yellow capsicum, cut into 4cm pieces

1 large red onion, halved, cut into thin wedges

2 tablespoons extra-virgin olive oil

250g punnet cherry tomatoes

6 garlic cloves, unpeeled

1 tablespoon balsamic vinegar

1/2 cup fresh basil leaves, chopped

METHOD

STEP 1

Preheat oven to 180C/160C fan-forced.

STEP 2

Place zucchinis, pumpkin, capsicum, onion and oil in a large roasting pan. Season well with salt and pepper. Toss to combine.

STEP 3

Roast for 20 minutes. Add tomatoes and garlic. Toss to combine. Roast for a further 15 to 20 minutes or until vegetables are golden and tender.

STEP 4

Remove garlic from pan. Carefully squeeze garlic from skins and place in a small bowl. Using a fork, whisk in vinegar. Season with salt and pepper.

STEP 5

Using a potato masher, gently crush tomatoes in pan. Add basil and garlic dressing to vegetables. Toss gently to combine. Serve.

NUTRITION VALUE	781 KJ Energy, 9.9g fat, 1.3g saturated fat, 5g fiber, 4.4g protein, 18.9g carbs.

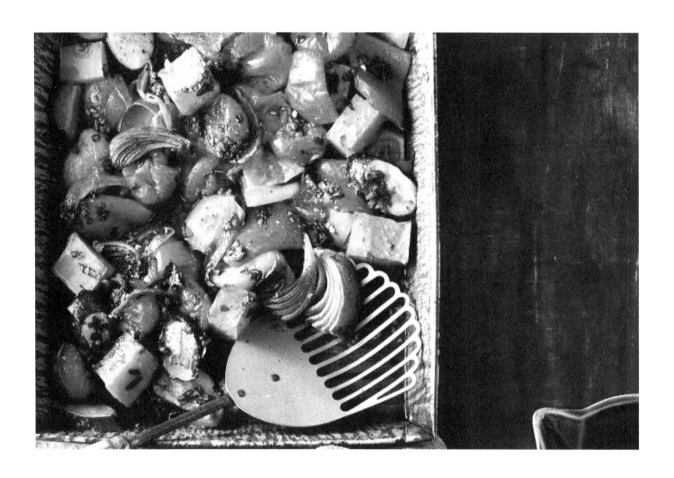

ROASTED VEGETABLE SALAD

With a hint of sweetness, this creamy citrus dressing plays well with lots of salads, including this roasted vegetable one.

INGREDIENTS

400g cauliflower, cut into florets

1 red capsicum, thickly sliced

400g kent pumpkin, peeled, cut into thin wedges

1 tablespoon extra-virgin olive oil

250 packet cooked whole baby beetroot, quartered

60g baby spinach

1/4 cup walnuts, toasted, chopped

2 tablespoons dried cranberries

2 teaspoons orange zest

ORANGE TAHINI AND MINT DRESSING
1/4 cup tahini

1 1/2 teaspoons orange rind, finely grated

2 tablespoons orange juice

2 tablespoons apple cider vinegar

1 teaspoon ground cumin

1 tablespoon fresh mint, finely chopped

METHOD

STEP 1
Preheat oven to 220C/200C fan-forced. Line a large baking tray with baking paper.

STEP 2
Place cauliflower, capsicum and pumpkin in a bowl. Drizzle with oil. Season well with salt and pepper. Toss to combine. Transfer to prepared tray, spreading vegetables to form a single layer.

STEP 3
Roast for 20 minutes or until vegetables are browned and tender. Cool for 10 minutes.

STEP 4
Meanwhile make the Orange, Tahini and Mint dressing; Place tahini, orange rind and juice, vinegar, cumin and mint in a jug. Season with salt and pepper. Stir to combine. Set aside.

STEP 5
Transfer vegetables to a bowl. Add beetroot, spinach, walnuts and cranberries. Drizzle salad with dressing and sprinkle with orange zest and mint leaves. Serve.

NUTRITION VALUE

1326 KJ Energy, 20.3g fat, 2.2g saturated fat, 8.1g fiber, 9.8g protein, 21.8g carbs.

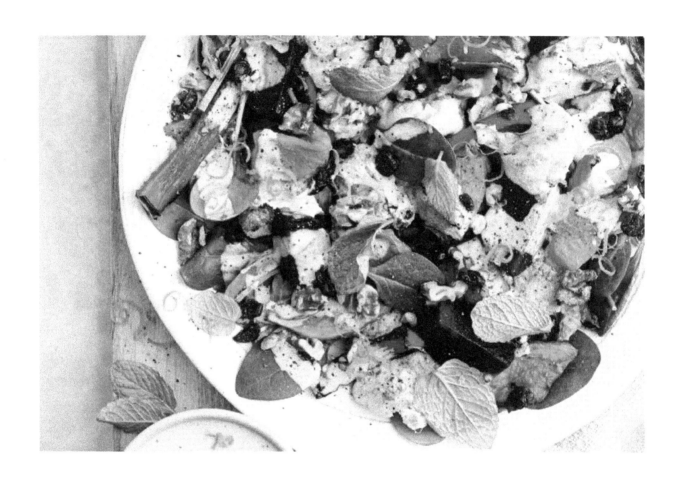

SAUTEED POTATOES IN GARLIC OIL

Spend that extra time with this recipe and create crispy golden potato bites that will spectacularly complement any roast dinner.

MAKES 8 SERVING/ TOTAL TIME 1 HOUR 20 MINUTE

INGREDIENTS

150ml peanut oil

8 large garlic cloves, peeled, thinly sliced

1kg Sebago potatoes, peeled, cut into 3-4cm pieces

Handful fresh sage leaves

METHOD

STEP 1

Heat the oil in a small saucepan over very low heat until shimmering. Add the garlic. Cook, over a very low heat, for 20 minutes or until golden and crisp but not burnt. Use a slotted spoon to transfer the garlic to a plate lined with paper towel to drain. Strain the oil through a fine sieve into a jug, repeating to remove all sediment.

STEP 2

Boil the potato in a saucepan of lightly salted boiling water for 12-15 minutes or until just tender. Drain. Refresh under cold running water. Set aside to cool and dry. Heat 80ml (1/3 cup) of the garlic oil in a large frying pan over medium heat. Cook the potato, in 2 batches, stirring frequently, for 10-15 minutes or until crisp and golden. Use a slotted spoon to transfer to a warmed plate.

STEP 3

Wipe the pan clean with paper towel. Add a little more oil to the pan over high heat and fry the sage leaves for a few seconds until crisp. Stir in the garlic and drizzle over the potato. Season.

NUTRITION VALUE	1190 KJ Energy, 8.7g fat, 1.9g saturated fat, 13.6g fiber, 11.3g protein, 32.2g carbs.

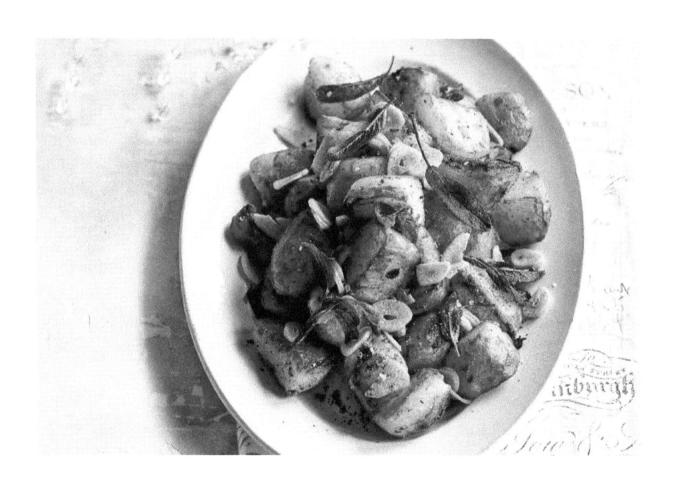

SPICY BLACK BEAN AND CORN SOUP WITH CHILLI

This spicy, satisfying vegetarian soup has a creamy texture and is rich in protein and fiber, thanks to the black beans.

MAKES 4 SERVING/ TOTAL TIME 8 HOUR 30 MINUTE

INGREDIENTS

220g (1 cup) dried black beans, rinsed, drained

2 teaspoons extra-virgin olive oil

1 large brown onion, finely chopped

2 celery sticks, finely chopped

2 garlic cloves, crushed

2 teaspoons ground cumin

2 teaspoons sweet paprika

1/2 teaspoon chili flakes

400g can crushed tomatoes

1.25L (5 cups) water

300g sweet potato, peeled, chopped

1 large sweet corn cob, kernels removed

2 tablespoons fresh coriander leaves, chopped

1 long fresh green chili, deseeded, finely chopped

METHOD

STEP 1
Place black beans in a large saucepan. Cover with enough cold water to come 5cm above beans. Bring to the boil over medium high heat. Cook for 10 minutes. Drain well.

STEP 2
Meanwhile, heat oil in a large non-stick frying pan over medium heat. Cook onion and celery, stirring, for 5 minutes or until soft. Add garlic, cumin, paprika and chili. Cook, stirring, for 1 minute or until aromatic.

STEP 3
Place onion mixture, beans, tomato and water in a large (6L) slow cooker. Cover. Cook on low for 7 hours. Add sweet potato and corn. Cover. Cook for a further 1 hour or until potato is tender and soup is thick. Season.

STEP 4
Combine coriander and green chili in a bowl. Divide soup among bowls. Top with coriander mixture. Serve with lime.

NUTRITION VALUE

1453 KJ Energy, 14g fat, 2g saturated fat, 17g fiber, 21g protein, 29g carbs.

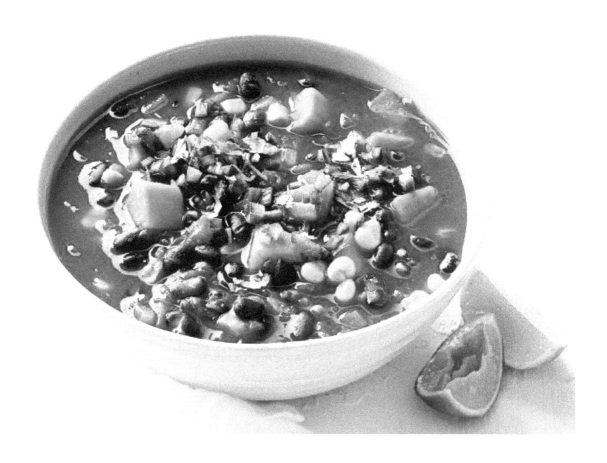

AYURVEDIC BEETROOT CURRY

Increase your vitality and health and tuck into this tasty curry tonight!

MAKES 4 SERVING/ TOTAL TIME 1 HOUR 50 MINUTE

INGREDIENTS

1.5kg beetroot, peeled, cut into 3cm cubes

2 tablespoons fresh ginger, grated

3 garlic cloves, crushed

2 teaspoons garam masala

2 teaspoons ground cumin

1 teaspoon ground coriander

1 teaspoon ground turmeric

400g can coconut cream

2 tablespoons coconut oil

2 brown onions, thinly sliced

4 sprigs fresh curry leaves

400g can chickpeas, drained, rinsed

1/3 cup red lentils, rinsed, drained

100g baby spinach

1 tablespoon lemon juice

Sprigs coriander, to serve

METHOD

STEP 1

Combine beetroot, ginger, garlic, spices and coconut cream in a large bowl. Toss to coat.

STEP 2

Heat coconut oil in a large saucepan over high heat. Cook onion and curry leaves, stirring, for 5 minutes or until well browned. Add beetroot mixture, chickpeas, lentils and 1 cup water. Season and stir to combine. Bring to the boil. Reduce heat to low and cook, covered, for 1 hour 15 minutes or until lentils and beetroot are tender. Stir in spinach and lemon juice. Serve sprinkled with coriander.

NUTRITION VALUE

2696 KJ Energy, 32.9g fat, 27.3g saturated fat, 21.6g fiber, 19.3g protein, 76.4g carbs.

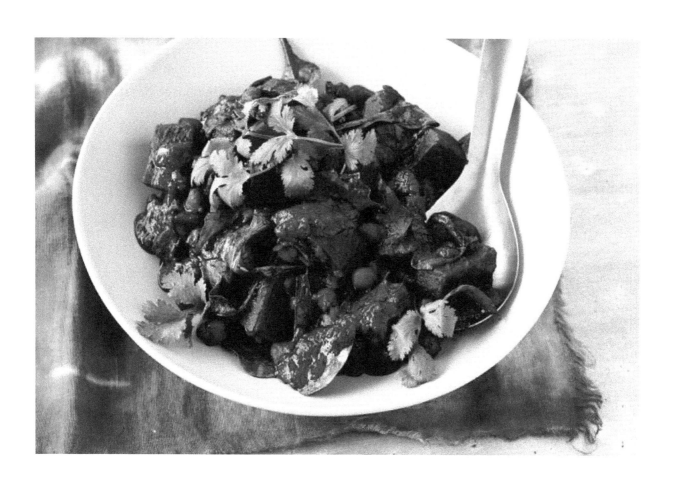

LENTIL, SPINACH & TOMATO SALAD

Recipe that everyone loves!

MAKES 4 SERVING/ TOTAL TIME 15 MINUTE

INGREDIENTS

2 x 400g cans brown lentils, rinsed, drained

4 ripe tomatoes, coarsely chopped

80g baby spinach leaves

100g flat beans, topped, cut into 2cm lengths diagonally

2 carrots, peeled, coarsely chopped

2 Lebanese cucumbers, coarsely chopped

1/2 cup chopped fresh continental parsley

1 tablespoon fresh lemon juice

1 tablespoon balsamic vinegar

1 tablespoon extra-virgin olive oil

1 garlic clove, crushed

Sliced crusty bread, to serve

METHOD

STEP 1

Place the lentils, tomato, spinach, beans, carrot, cucumber and parsley in a large bowl and gently toss until just combined.

STEP 2

Use a balloon whisk to whisk together the lemon juice, vinegar, oil and garlic in a small bowl. Season with pepper.

STEP 3

Drizzle the dressing over the salad and toss until well combined. Divide the salad among serving bowls. Serve with crusty bread.

NUTRITION VALUE

800 KJ Energy, 5g fat, 1g saturated fat, 10g fiber, 12g protein, 19g carbs.

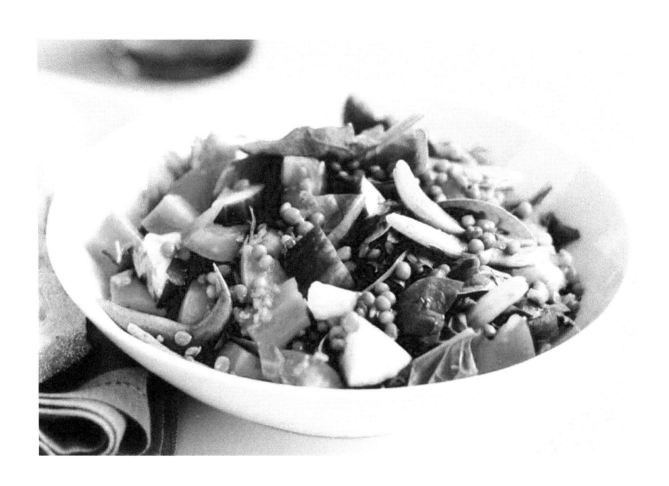

BROWN RICE AND HARISSA ROASTED VEGETABLE SALAD

This colorful salad incorporates all our favorite roast vegetables with tasty brown rice and spicy harissa.

MAKES 4 SERVING/ TOTAL TIME 45 MINUTE

INGREDIENTS

1 cup medium-grain brown rice, rinsed

1 medium red capsicum, chopped

1 medium yellow capsicum, chopped

1/2 small orange sweet potato, thinly sliced

2 small zucchinis, halved, chopped

2 baby eggplant, halved, chopped

1 tablespoon harissa

1/4 cup extra-virgin olive oil

2 teaspoons finely grated lemon rind

2 tablespoons lemon juice

1 tablespoon chopped fresh oregano leaves

fresh oregano leaves, to serve

METHOD

STEP 1

Preheat oven to 220°C/ 200°C fan-forced. Cook rice in a large saucepan of boiling, salted water, following packet directions, until tender. Drain.

STEP 2

Meanwhile, place capsicum, potato, zucchinis, eggplant, harissa and 1 tablespoon oil in a roasting pan. Toss to combine. Roast for 20 minutes or until vegetables are tender.

STEP 3

Place rice, capsicum mixture, remaining oil, lemon rind, lemon juice and oregano in a large bowl. Season with salt and pepper. Toss to combine. Top with oregano leaves. Serve.

NUTRITION VALUE

1439 KJ Energy, 16g fat, 3g saturated fat, 4g fiber, 5g protein, 44g carbs.

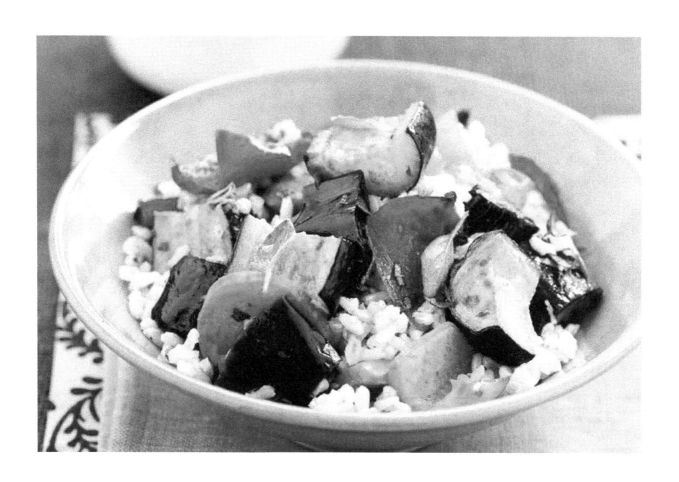

ORANGE SALAD

Make the most of oranges at the peak of their season in this sensational salad.

MAKES 6 SERVING/ TOTAL TIME 10 MINUTE

INGREDIENTS

4 large oranges, peeled, pith removed and discarded, sliced into 2cm rounds

1 red onion, finely sliced

3 tablespoons finely chopped flat-leaf parsley

1/4 cup (60ml) olive oil

1 tablespoon orange juice

2 teaspoons orange blossom water*

2 tablespoons slivered pistachios, to serve

METHOD
STEP 1

Lay oranges on a platter. Sprinkle with onion and parsley. Combine oil, juice and blossom water and season. Dress salad just before serving and season with freshly ground pepper. Garnish with nuts.

NUTRITION VALUE

516 KJ Energy, 8g fat, 1g saturated fat, 3g fiber, 2g protein, 9g carbs.

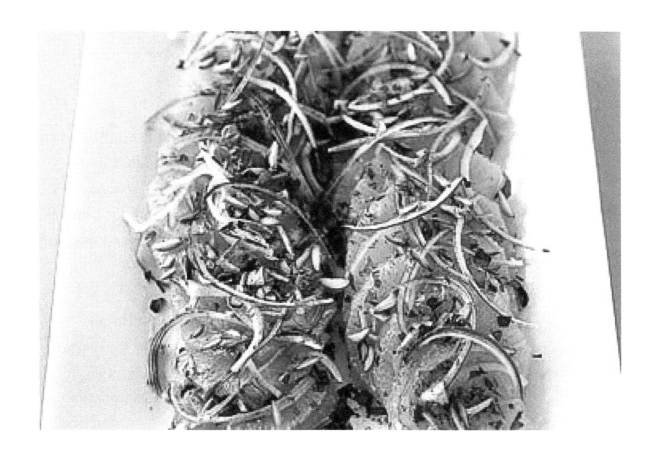

MOROCCAN PUMPKIN SOUP

Take an Australian classic like pumpkin soup, add a Moroccan twist and make this "souper" meal which is vegan friendly.

MAKES 6 SERVING/ TOTAL TIME 1 HOUR 25 MINUTE

INGREDIENTS

1/4 cup (60ml) olive oil

1 leek, white part only, thinly sliced

3 cloves garlic, finely chopped

1 red birdseye chili, finely chopped

1 cinnamon stick

3cm piece ginger, peeled, thinly sliced

1 1/2 teaspoons cumin seeds

2 carrots, peeled, coarsely chopped

1.5kg butternut or Queensland blue pumpkin, peeled, seeded cut into 3cm pieces

1/3 cup (70g) yellow split peas

Juice of 1/2 lemon

Coriander sprigs, to serve

Soup sprinkles, to serve

METHOD

STEP 1

Heat oil in a large saucepan over low-medium heat and cook leek, garlic and 2 teaspoons salt, stirring occasionally, for 3 minutes or until soft. Add chili, cinnamon, ginger and cumin and stir for 1 minute or until fragrant. Add carrots, pumpkin and split peas. Stir to coat in onion mixture.

STEP 2

Add 1.5 liters water to saucepan and bring to the boil, then simmer for 50 minutes or until split peas are soft.

STEP 3

Remove and discard cinnamon stick from soup. Add lemon juice then process or blend soup, in small batches, in a food processor or blender until smooth. Return soup to pan and reheat over medium heat. Serve topped with coriander sprigs and soup sprinkles.

NUTRITION VALUE	1066 KJ Energy, 11g fat, 2g saturated fat, 8g fiber, 9g protein, 26g carbs.

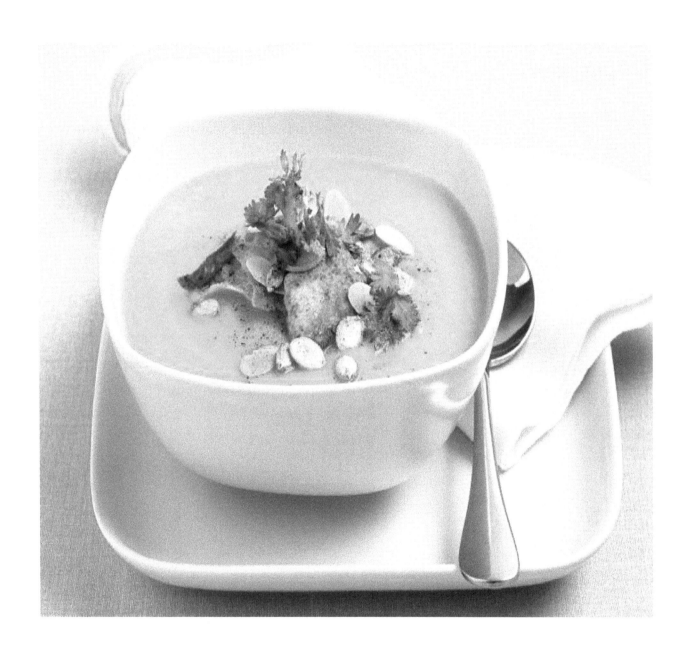

LENTIL SOUP

This old favorite is best served with chunks of crusty bread to mop up every last skerrick.

MAKES 4 SERVING/ TOTAL TIME 35 MINUTE

INGREDIENTS

1 tablespoon olive oil

1 brown onion, finely chopped

1 carrot, peeled, finely chopped

1 celery stick, trimmed, finely chopped

2 x 400g cans brown lentils, rinsed, drained

400g can diced tomatoes

500ml (2 cups) Massel vegetable liquid stock

2 dried bay leaves

2 teaspoons dried oregano leaves

1/4 cup chopped fresh continental parsley

Olive oil (optional), to drizzle

25g (1/3 cup) finely grated parmesan

METHOD

STEP 1

Heat the oil in a large saucepan over medium heat. Cook onion, carrot and celery, stirring occasionally, for 5 minutes or until soft. Stir in lentils, tomato, stock, bay leaves and oregano. Reduce heat to low. Simmer for 10 minutes or until mixture reduces slightly. Set aside for 5 minutes to cool. Remove and discard the bay leaves.

STEP 2

Process half the soup in a food processor until smooth. Return to the pan. Cook, stirring, over medium heat until heated through. Stir in the parsley.

STEP 3

Divide among serving bowls. Drizzle over oil, if desired. Top with parmesan.

NUTRITION VALUE

867 KJ Energy, 8g fat, 2g saturated fat, 8g fiber, 13g protein, 17g carbs.

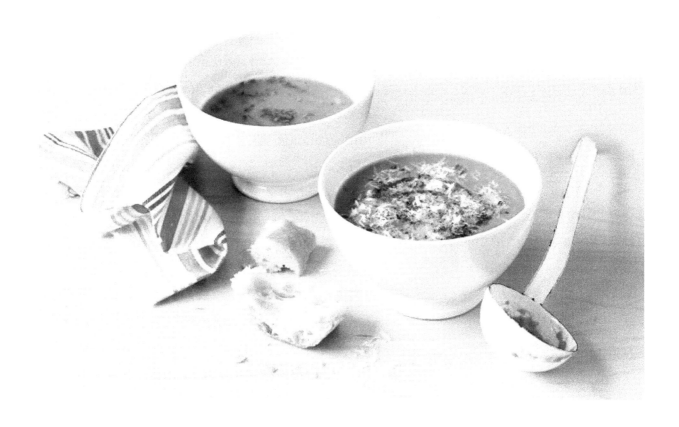

SPINACH DHAL WITH GARLIC BREAD

A satisfying **vegan** meal of tasty lentils served with warm and delicious garlic bread.

MAKES 4 SERVING/ TOTAL TIME 30 MINUTE

INGREDIENTS

1 tablespoon olive oil

1 brown onion, halved, finely chopped

8 baby desiree potatoes, quartered

1 teaspoon ground cumin

1 teaspoon ground coriander

500ml (2 cups) water

1 tablespoon tomato paste

1 x 400g can brown lentils, rinsed, drained

80g baby spinach leaves

GARLIC BREAD

2 pieces (22cm-diameter) Lebanese bread

1 tablespoon olive oil

2 garlic cloves, crushed

METHOD

STEP 1

Preheat oven to 180°C. Heat the oil in a saucepan over medium heat. Add the onion and potato and cook, stirring, for 5 minutes or until the onion is soft. Add the cumin and coriander and cook, stirring, for 1 minute or until aromatic.

STEP 2

Add the water and tomato paste and bring to the boil. Reduce heat to medium and simmer, stirring occasionally, for 10 minutes or until liquid reduces by half.

STEP 3

Meanwhile, to make the garlic bread, place the bread on a baking tray. Combine the oil and garlic in a small bowl. Brush both sides of the bread evenly with garlic mixture. Season with salt. Bake for 8 minutes or until crisp. Break into wedges.

STEP 4

Add the lentils to the potato mixture and cook for 2 minutes or until heated through. Add spinach and stir until just wilted. Season with salt and pepper.

NUTRITION VALUE

1585 KJ Energy, 8g fat, 1g saturated fat, 9g fiber, 14g protein, 63g carbs.

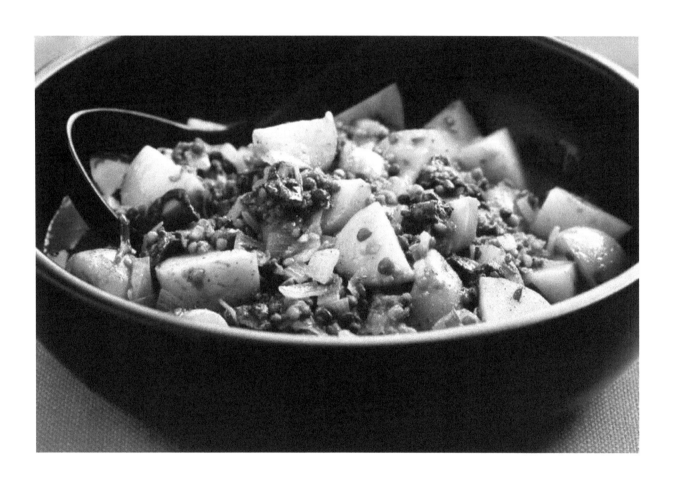

ASIAN-STYLE CURRIED VEGETABLE BROTH

Create a richly flavorsome curry soup using tofu, rice noodles and a handful of fresh ingredients.

MAKES 4 SERVING/ TOTAL TIME 30 MINUTE

INGREDIENTS

1/4 cup green curry paste

320g packet nigari tofu (extra firm), cut into 2cm cubes

150ml light coconut milk

2 cups Massel vegetable liquid stock

2 1/2 cups water

80g dried rice vermicelli noodles

1 bunch gai plum, stalks diagonally sliced, leaves shredded

125g packet fresh baby corn, halved lengthways

Coriander leaves, to serve

METHOD

STEP 1

Heat curries paste in a large wok over medium heat, stirring, for 1 to 2 minutes, or until aromatic. Add tofu. Cook, tossing gently, for 1 minute. Add coconut milk, stock and water. Bring to a simmer.

STEP 2

Add noodles and gai lum stalks to wok. Cook for 5 minutes, or until noodles are almost tender.

STEP 3

Add gai lum leaves and corn to wok. Cook for 2 to 3 minutes, or until leaves wilt. Divide broth between 4 serving bowls. Top with coriander. Serve.

NUTRITION VALUE

100KJ Energy, 13.6g fat, 2.5g saturated fat, 6g fiber, 14.6g protein, 23.8g carbs.

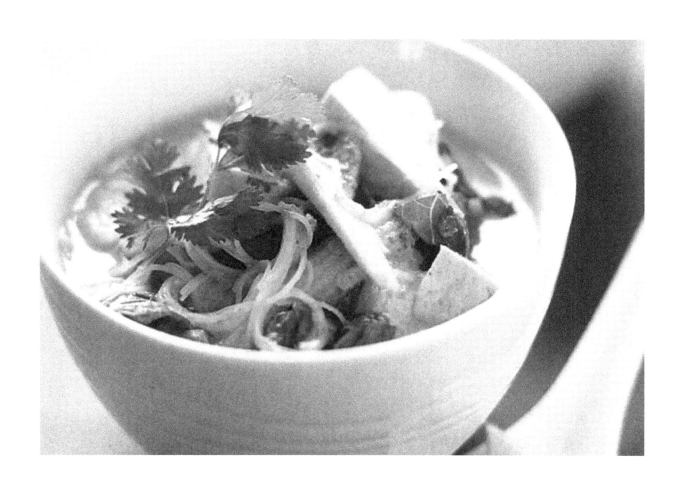

Lightning Source UK Ltd.
Milton Keynes UK
UKHW051844030521
383069UK00006B/132